# TheWaikikiDiet

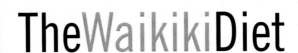

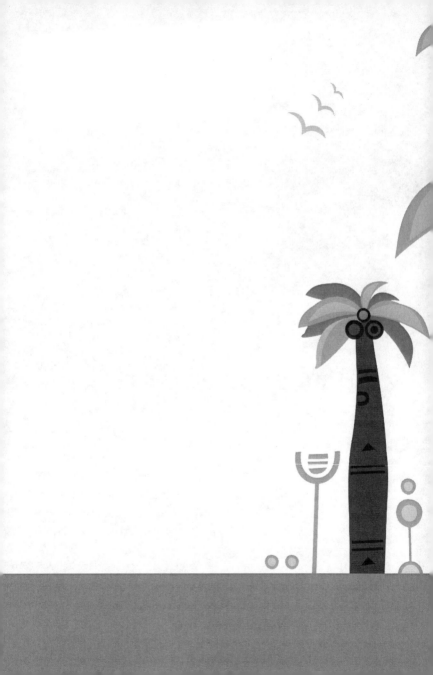

A Journey to Weight Loss, Health, Physical Exercise,
the History of Captain Cook, and the Hawaiian Royalty

Marianne DeVries

# TheWaikikiDiet

TATE PUBLISHING & Enterprises

Published by Tate Publishing & Enterprises, LLC
127 E. Trade Center Terrace | Mustang, Oklahoma 73064 USA
1.888.361.9473 | www.tatepublishing.com

Tate Publishing is committed to excellence in the publishing industry. The company reflects the philosophy established by the founders, based on Psalm 68:11,
*"The Lord gave the word and great was the company of those who published it."*

Book design copyright © 2008 by Tate Publishing, LLC. All rights reserved.
*Cover design by Stephanie Woloszyn*
*Interior design by Kellie Southerland*

Published in the United States of America

ISBN: 978-1-60604-184-0
1. Health & Fitness: Diets: Better Health & Weight Loss
2. History: State: Hawaii
08.06.17

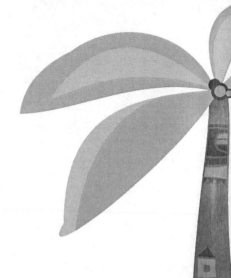

# Dedication

I dedicate this book to my Lord and Savior, family, friends, and anyone who needs a well-balanced diet to lose excess weight or to make healthier food choices that will increase the quality of life. I also dedicate this book to the people of Hawaii with *aloha*. I sincerely hope that this book will be a blessing to you.

# Acknowledgements

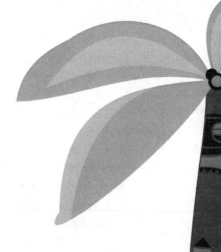

This book would not have come together without the help of many people. A special thanks to the founder of Tate Publishing, Dr. Richard Tate, who believed in the content of the book and the wonderful staff at Tate Publishing, who worked with me to get this book to you, the reader.

Thanks to my sons, Francisco and Frankie, who did not stop believing in my creative abilities and dreams. The sweetness of Frankie would not let me call myself fat—just chubby. And dear Francisco would encourage me to exercise, and no matter my weight he continued to lift me like a bag of potatoes.

I am grateful for mother's cooking. Low-calorie gourmet meals and my dad's vegetable garden produced pesticide-free, delicious veggies. Thanks to my parents for their continued support.

Thanks to my friends—Joyce Sheppard, Lisa Boyd, Mitzi Sullivan, Dr. Rinia Wijngaarde, Melissa (my daughter-in-law to be), and my auntie Carmen—for their encouragement.

In memory of my late pastor, Dr. D. James Kennedy. Thank you for giving to the Lord, I am a life that was changed.

Of course, the greatest thanks and glory goes to Jesus Christ, God Almighty, whose hand I can trace in my life and who made this book possible.

# Table of Contents

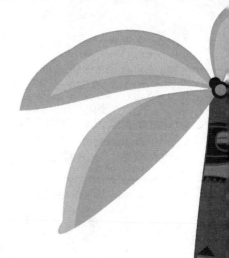

# Foreword

This book truly takes the reader on a real and spiritual journey to some of the most important places in life, self-discovery, and health. My dear friend, Marianne, takes you along with her to beautiful Hawaii. You feel as though you are right there with her, experiencing her excitement and happiness as she emotionally and physically triumphs over her "chubbiness." As she felt so much better about herself, she was more open to enjoying the sights and senses around her—like the sweet Hawaiian music, the color of the water, and the scents of the tropical flowers. The pain of struggling to lose weight was behind her, and this opened a myriad of new portals for her to experience.

Like many of us, including myself, Marianne tried many crash diets that led only to a temporary fix then demoralization as the pounds always crept back onto her body. As explained in this book, we need to take a look at the emotions that cause us to overeat. This is the beginning of a permanent healing and new way of life. Marianne shares her success with us by explaining the steps she took in a clear and concise way, so that others can easily follow her lead. Once you start to read the book, you will see clearly what I mean. Knowledge is power that will set you free in many ways.

*The Waikiki Diet* offers much more to everyone than a road to losing weight. It outlines a spiritual path that can be taken not only by someone wishing to lose weight, but also by anyone aspiring to a better way of life. Daily motivations and affirmations combined with healthy eating and exercise will benefit any reader. I hope you will enjoy and be enriched as much as I was by Marianne's book.

I felt I was sitting under the banyan tree with Marianne and her friend in Hawaii while I was reading the history of the Hawaiian Royalty. I could envisage the lovely Hawaiian woman, Moana, verbally recounting the stories, to the group seated around her, in the beautifully written history of Hawaii Marianne has captured and put into this book. Captain Cook's adventures and misadventures intrigued me. I found the tribal customs of that era interesting along with the arrival of the missionaries from America. What an amazing history for a small group of islands in the middle of the Pacific Ocean!

I met Marianne about twenty years ago when we were both working in the tourist industry. She began working part time with us as she had other interests, but soon she became the manager of the office. Always dedicated and caring, Marianne was very popular and a great leader. She stood up for what was right, seeking to encourage and teach her staff. As a good and very religious person, we always knew we could trust her. Marianne then moved to another company, and it was not long before I was working at the same place. I have known Marianne for many years and have seen how she does nice, thoughtful things for others and myself, never even telling us about it or expecting any thanks. Follow her suggestions given with love from a caring heart, and you will see where the contents of this book will take you.

Lisa Boyd
*Artist*

# Introduction

I have won the battle. I have lost forty pounds before my trip to Hawaii. It was quite a feat, but I struggled to make it happen. The diet plan effective for me consisted of:

1. smaller portions
2. frequent meals every three hours
3. a daily calorie allowance
4. cutting fat, sugar, and carbohydrates
5. nutritional and healthy choices

6. cutting diet drinks
7. exercise, walking, biking, and working out at the gym
8. having a support buddy
9. prayer—God's help
10. reading Bible verses
11. daily motivation

Losing weight for obese people is one of the hardest things to do. Usually the weight loss problem has a deeper connection with emotions. Before pursuing a weight-loss program, the emotional issues need to be dealt with so the diet will have a chance to succeed.

I struggled with weight loss for many years (forty-plus). I have studied, tried, and followed so many different diets. I even joined several weight-loss programs and ordered their food, but I was not successful in sticking to the programs. However, I acquired more and more nutritional information that became useful to me in choosing a diet that would eventually be effective and be easy to follow.

Because of the effectiveness of this diet plan—and to help others with their weight problems—I felt compelled to write this book to share my diet, exercise plan, and methods.

The program blends so well with my daily life, it probably would do the same for many obese people.

Running around with an overweight body had serious effects on my health. My physician recommended, after seeing my lab test result with a high LDL and triglycerides levels and my blood pressure still elevated, that I should lose weight. I had more fat then muscle, which created an unhealthy body composition. I started exercising to lose fat and retain muscle, which resulted in a healthier body composition. After five months of diet and exercise, my lab test results did indeed come back with much lower numbers. Needless to say, both my physician and I were ecstatic with the positive results.

I am sure you can do what I did. Just copy me, and— *voila!*—the pounds will fall off.

Remember that weight loss is a journey. If you get to your ideal weight, you have reached your destination— however, the journey is not over. The new weight and body composition have to be kept and maintained .You can't say, "I did it, now goodbye, Charlie," and then go back to your old ways of eating. You will have to keep making the right nutritional choices, as well lowering your caloric intake and ingesting smaller portions.

God Bless,
Marianne

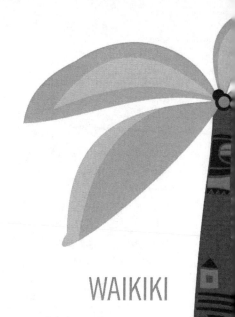

# WAIKIKI

I was so excited to have reached my target weight for my Hawaiian trip. My efforts and perseverance had paid off. I lost forty pounds in five-and-a-half months by following a simple diet and exercise plan.

*Aloha*! Maggie and I found a table on the busy Duke's Canoe Club[1] terrace of our hotel overlooking the beach and the Pacific Ocean. A soft breeze stirred the air, and the sun would be setting soon—the sky was getting a spectacular orange and yellow glow. We arrived about four hours ago at Honolulu airport, picked up a car, and made our way to the hotel on Waikiki. We both wanted something small to eat and decided to share a tuna melt sandwich. Wow! That had quite some calories, but since we decided to share it, calories would be cut in half. We are both women over forty and have to watch our caloric and fat intake. Maggie ordered two virgin Mai Tai drinks for us. I was watching the activity on the beach and the surfers who were trying to catch waves before it got dark. It was a gorgeous, peaceful evening. The torches on the beach were lit, and soft music came from the terrace next door. Three guys playing instruments and a female vocalist under the banyan tree sang popular Hawaiian songs like "Tiny Bubbles" and "Blue Hawaii." The server came with the drinks, which we sipped quickly. The sandwich was delicious and we gobbled it up. We paid the bill and then walked on the sandy beach to the hotel next door where we stood for a while listening to the sweet Hawaiian music.

We cut through to the sidewalk where the entertainment for the tourists was going on; we heard a voice of a young girl, probably seven or eight years old, singing. She attracted many tourists with her angelic voice. Her dad controlled the PA system, and in front of the system was a basket for tips. She was quite a natural performer and her tip bucket was steadily becoming full. Men painted themselves entirely in gold or silver and pretended to be statues. Tourists stood and posed in pictures with these statues. Maggie and I continued to walk down the sidewalk, purchasing two leis at the stand underneath the humongous banyan tree at the International Market Place. The leis, made of fresh white and pink plumeria flowers, engulfed our olfactory senses with their beautiful aroma every time a gust of wind blew by us. Also, we each got a flower for our hair. I was told to wear mine on the right side since I am single, and Maggie had to wear hers on the left side since she was married. We walked around for another half hour looking at the windows of the different stores and at the myriad of performers. Before calling it quits for the evening, we hopped in an ABC store, across from our hotel, where we bought two small pouches of Hawaiian dark chocolates and a container of cold pineapple chunks.

Famished after a good night's sleep, we went for breakfast at the Hula Girl[2], which overlooked the ocean. We were greeted with a big *aloha* and a warm smile. The sun shone brightly and the ocean had a gorgeous aqua-turquoise shade. The tourists were looking for a spot on the beach to settle in for the day. Colorful cabanas and loungers were already placed on the sand and under the palm trees. The surfers were out in the water, actively pursuing waves. I enjoyed a Bikini omelet made of egg white, spinach, and cheese. No bread, just a slice of pineapple, which I topped with half a spoon of coconut syrup. A hot cup of decaf coffee complimented this scrumptious low-calorie breakfast. "*ai ono*" delicious food.

After breakfast we drove to the north shore of Oahu. We took the Pali (cliff) Highway, that cuts through the most majestic tree lined Koolau Mountain Range to the windward (northeast) side of Oahu with spectacular ocean views, to get to the coastline highway. We enjoyed melodious music from the famous Hawaiian singer, IZ coming from the car radio. His renditions of "Somewhere Over The Rainbow/What A Wonderful World" and "n Dis Life" were just beautiful. What a talent! We made a quick stop at the Byodo-In Buddist Temple at the foot of the Koolau mountains in the Valley of the Temples. The temple is a replica of the Byodo-In in Uji, Japan. We traveled further to the macadamia nut farm. At the farm store we were invited to taste the variety of macadamia nut coffees. While sipping the coffee I noticed the American flag against the wall; underneath was a sign saying, " One Nation under God, In Whom We Trust." It was heartwarming to see that. Two local artists shared that room displaying their merchandise—watercolor paintings of Hawaii and jewelry. Next we were invited to sample the macadamia nuts with flavors such as plain, onion & chives, and cinnamon. The milk and dark chocolate-covered macadamia nuts were just yummy. With the added calories we drove a bit farther to the Kualoa Ranch where we got lost in the gift shop. We watched two horses being affectionate. Playfully kissing each other. That was an amazing site that made me realize that God has favor on animals too. Another thing that I realized was that I have not seen overweight horses. I guess their lifestyle is much more active than ours is, and their food intake is controlled by the caretaker. How disciplined are we in our food intake and other areas of our lives? Are we strong or weak, do we struggle, or are we a combination of all three at certain times?

We followed the coastline highway farther north to the tip of the North Shore with its charming towns. The North Shore is the popular area for pro surfers because of the huge, dangerous waves. We continued making our way back to Waikiki and stopped en route at the Dole Plantation for a pineapple ice cream. We each got a cone for the road and moved on enjoying the magnificent mountain and ocean views as well as the delicious ice cream. Back in Waikiki we walked over to the Moana Surfrider hotel and settled in one of the chairs underneath the banyan tree overlooking the blue ocean. At the table next to us was Moana, a beautiful Hawaiian lady with a purple orchid in her long dark hair. We listened to her conversation with a group of tourists. Her voice was enchanting as she shared a few native recipes with them. One of the tourists asked if she could show them a few hula steps, which she gladly did. She jumped up, put her feet together, her knees slightly bent, and started swaying to the right and to the left. She raised her arms up, and made a "U" motion. The tourists copied her, and they seemed to have so much fun. She invited them to come back tomorrow midday for stories about the intriguing Captain Cook and the Hawaiian royalty.

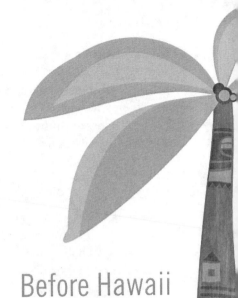

# Before Hawaii

It was the day after New Year's, January the second. I thought, *Gosh, all the Christmas parties during the month of December surely added pounds to my body* as I stood in front of the mirror. I did not look *that* fat, but why did I feel fat? And why did I have to get a bigger dress and pant size? Why was I hiding from any person who wanted to snap a picture of me? I was definitely gaining weight, but I could not see nor did I want to see it when I looked in the mirror. I sucked my cheeks in so that I would not look too round and fat. I felt heavy and unhealthy. I had high blood pressure, and even with medicine it was slightly elevated. It was time to do something about it. I hated the idea of high blood-pressure and cholesterol pills for the rest of my life, and who knew what other pills would be added in the years to come. Consequently, having to deal with the side effects of the medication did not paint a pretty picture. The first thing I did was to go shopping for a scale.

What a shock to see my weight displayed on the scale—210 pounds. "Wow! That's crazy," I said aloud as soon as I stepped off the scale. I picked up literature about weight-loss diets to decide which to follow. I was always chubby and had been on and off diets most of my life. I often underwent crash diets that had quick results; however, the weight always came back once I was off the diet. I knew this time I could not go on a crash diet; I was determined to make the weight loss permanent. I knew that six meals a day was the healthiest thus the best way to go. It included all the food groups. The diet I selected was based on smaller portions, low-fat and low-sugar intake—as well as healthier choices, increased my fiber intake such as whole grain products instead of white bread, white rice, and white pasta with little or no nutritional benefits. The diet included decaffeinated coffee with half-&-half fat-free cream, no sugar, twice a day. It was simple and easy to follow. Actually, it was a dream diet. I started dropping two to three pounds a week. In addition to the diet plan, I went biking in my neighborhood. I started with fifteen minutes daily and then gradually increased to forty minutes once or twice a day. I did some stretching exercises and weight training with five-pound dumbbells. At times I did not feel like exercising, but I had to push myself. After only ten minutes of biking, I would feel great and be so energized that the forty minutes were done with no effort.

The first ten pounds were off in three weeks, and it was a great feeling. The fat was melting, and everyday I was feeling better.

I had lost already nineteen pounds when the diet was put on hold for the Sunday before President's Day since we were celebrating with friends. I enjoyed the calorie-rich homemade appetizers, main course, and desserts, although I only ate small portions. I was very aware of the calories that I was taking in. With every bite a voice told me, "Here … more calories than you are supposed to have," then another voice said, "Hey, the host might be insulted, I better take another bite." I knew I would pay for the consequences of that rich food. I definitely had a setback. I had to start again after that weekend and get rid of the added calories. If I only had taken one lone bite of the rich food, I probably would not have gained weight.

My days started with an egg-white omelet stuffed with a slice of fat-free melted Swiss cheese, two vegetables, one slice of whole-grain toast (no butter); half a glass of V8; a wedge of pineapple, papaya, or apple; and a cup of decaf coffee. I am a coffee drinker; if you aren't, you may have hot tea or iced tea. But no more than two cups of decaf coffee a day.

I snacked once between lunch and dinner. Actually I was eating all day long; however, it was all healthy, low-calorie food. Most important of all, my blood-sugar level did not drop.

Before my new way of eating, I had started the day with a cup of regular coffee; around ten o'clock in the morning I would have another cup with a few bites of cake, a donut, a bagel, or whatever was brought in and left in the office kitchen for the staff to eat. Most of the time for lunch, the food was a quick bite of whatever fast food was picked up by a coworker and another cup of coffee for an energy boost. Between three and five in the afternoon was my desperate time; my energy level was so low, I had to eat anything to be able to function. I needed food and grabbed whatever I could get my hands on—like chocolate, chips, and cookies to lift me up. All that bad stuff I consumed. My body stored fat instead of burning it. I was dehydrated because I did not drink enough water during the day.

My energy was out of whack, it went up and down during the day because my blood-sugar level did not stay constant due to not eating the proper nutritional snack and meal every three hours.

For dinner I had usually a frozen meal or sandwich. Most of the time I left work pretty late in the evening.

When I got home, it was a quick shower and straight to bed. I was living quite an unhealthy lifestyle with depleted nutritional reserves.

After six years of living this stressful, fast-paced, unhealthy, and unbalanced life, I decided to do something about it. I resigned from my position as General Manager and relocated; however, I stayed with the company working from home. This arrangement enabled me to pursue a new lifestyle. The first two months I was tempted by certain foods I saw in the fridge and on commercials and by the different restaurants I passed when on the road. I used to love going for coffee, a pastry, or a bagel. With God's help I was eventually able to switch off those temptations by focusing on the food that I was allowed for that day and making it gourmet and delicious in my mind.

On Sundays, I allowed myself to eat what I like. However, it would not be an *all I can eat, high-calorie day*. Smaller portions and calorie counting was still important on Sundays.

Holidays and trips came and went. The diet was put on hold during trips and then resumed again. However, I made sure I stayed on target with my weight loss. Days turned into months, and after five and a half months, I was forty pounds lighter and my body was nicely toned. Wow, amazing! I had reached my goal for my Hawaiian trip. It was fantastic that some of my old, smaller-size clothes in my closet were fitting again. I was very happy with the weight loss. It had just the desired weight that I wanted for my trip.

I looked and felt great, and I was getting so many compliments. The question always was "How did you lose the weight, and how did you tone your body?"

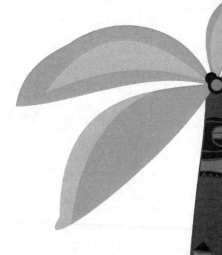

# Are You Ready for a Life Change?

## Reality

When will you start losing weight? What are you doing with your overweight body? Get on the wagon to weight loss, exercise, and healthy food. *Are you on?* Did you make a commitment to read this book and follow the diet plan for at least a period of time? *Just marvelous! Welcome onboard!*

## Where to start

> "In all human affairs there are efforts, and there are results, and the strength of the effort is the measure of the result."
>
> *James Allen*

Before you start dieting, you have to reprogram your mind by renewing it to overcome the temptations and to adopt this new way of eating. Be strong; stick to your diet. If you fail a day, pick it up again. Continue, keeping in mind the reason why you want to lose weight. Remember it is one day at a time. Give yourself a pat on the back before going to sleep. Tell yourself, "Self, you have done it today. Kudos." Tomorrow, do it again. You are actually choosing a new way of eating for life. Remember, it is a lifestyle change. Keep your focus on your purpose!

## The Mind

> "All that a man achieves and all that he fails to achieves is the direct result of his own thoughts."
>
> *James Allen*

In the mind thoughts are formed. Thoughts create emotions, which produce actions or behavior that could be good or bad, negative or positive, constructive or destructive. Get rid of bad thoughts. You should strive to have good thoughts, true and right ones. If you practice to have only positive thoughts about every aspect in your life, past, present, and future, as well as positive thoughts about people, you will get the right attitude.

A right attitude can conquer any challenge, trial, adversity, or failure that comes your way. The right attitude will make you a happy and content person. In order to do so, you have to change the way you think; you have to let go of negative, false, impure thoughts that dwell in your mind. Your mindset, conscious or subconscious, has a stronghold on your behavior and your habits, limiting you to change and move forward with the right attitude. It is easier to be disciplined and to develop good habits when you have the right attitude. Temptations begin in the mind. A way to resist it is to stay focused on your weight-loss goal and vision for your life and to quote scripture, saying, "It is written that ... " [see Bible verses in the chapter *Bible Verses and Songs*.]

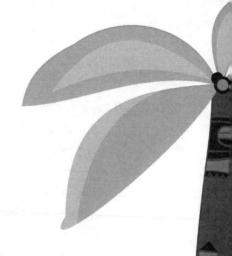

# First Things First

Buy a new notebook. Designate it for your new life-style. Paste a white sheet of paper on the front cover and write on it, "My Journey to Weight Loss, Exercise, and Health." On the bottom of the cover page, write your name and starting date.

The reason for this journal is to create your own personal profile and to record your nutritional information, weight-loss plan, preparation, and your successes, such as:

1. Who I am
2. How I see myself
3. Reasons to change
4. Weight-loss goals and target dates
5. Mindset struggles and the plan to overcome them
6. Daily menu plan
7. Important advice from my diet buddy
8. Weekly weight loss
9. Nutritional knowledge

The first area you must address before the weight loss will begin is the second section, How I See Myself. Write the following questions—feel free to add more!—then answer them. Fold your page in half. Write the questions on the left side of the page and your answer on right side.

> "For true success ask yourself these four questions: Why? Why not? Why not me? Why not now?"
>
> *James Allen*

1. Do I eat to stay alive and be healthy?
2. Do I overeat because the foods taste so good?

3. Do I eat to be comforted (emotions)?
4. Do I eat to feel good, to be pacified?
5. Do I like myself fat ? Why or why not?
6. Do I want to lose weight? Why should I or why shouldn't I?
7. Do I think that food controls me?
8. Why do I overeat?

## The Big Question

What do I have to do to get rid of old ways of thinking in order to overcome these obstacles and to stay focused and committed to the weight loss plan?

*Congrats on beginning the journey. Let's move on to weight-loss goals!*

1. *Why do I want to lose weight?* Write all the reasons. Most overweight people have more than one reason.

2. *How much do I want to lose?* Consider this carefully and realistically. Do research; find what your ideal weight should be—both medically and in accordance with your personal body structure.

3. *How long do I want to pursue this weight loss? What is my target date?* Do you have a particular date, month, or year in mind? For example, if you want to lose thirty pounds, do not write your target date two months from your start date. That will not work. Calculate about two pounds per week. When you lose two pounds steadily, you will not gain it back so fast. It is much healthier for your body than if you were on a crash diet where you lose six pounds per week, then gain that weight back within a day or two. Your sacrifice would be in vain.

4. *What physical exercise program do I want to do?* Walking, bicycling, weightlifting, swimming, playing tennis, jumping rope, hula dancing, taking aerobics, boxing, or joining a gym? Exercise benefits our overall health and is necessary for the body and mind. not only during this time but also for the rest of your life. Exercise[1] not only promotes weight loss, it strengthen our muscles and bones. It increases our lung capacity, and it aides to control blood sugar in diabetics by preventing sugar from accumulating in the blood. Exercise also

lowers the risk of heart disease, breast and colon cancers[41]. If you do not exercise, you could always walk. Get walking shoes and start. You could go to a park or walk in your neighborhood. If you have not exercised since you were in school or for a few years, or if you are really overweight, remember you have to start slow. Start to walk for fifteen minutes at your regular pace everyday. Do it in the morning (if you can) and afternoon. Remember to discuss your weight loss diet and exercise plan with your physician. After three days increase to twenty minutes; if you are up to it, go a little bit faster. If it is too much for you, slow down. Listen to your body. Eventually you should do thirty to forty minutes of brisk walking every day. If you join a gym, make sure that a physical trainer instructs you how, why, and how long to use the equipment, as well as what your heart-rate range should be when you do cardio exercises. Ask the trainer to give you a personal training plan. Be informed before you start working out.

## Support Buddy

> "The man who cannot endure to have his errors and shortcomings brought to the surface and made known, but tries to hide them, is unfit to walk the highway of truth."
> *James Allen*

You need a Support Buddy—which I refer to as a sup buddy—for this period of time. The sup buddy should be willing to commit to your entire diet period. It should be someone who wants you to succeed. A sincere and caring person will encourage you. You want someone who will be firm with you, who has your best interest at heart. Ask your prospective sup buddy the following questions:

1. Are you willing to listen to and discuss my feelings—such as fears, weaknesses, and strengths?

2. Are you willing to be called at least three times a day for encouragement; discussion of my achievements and setbacks; or when I get tempted and feel weak?

3. Are you willing to celebrate with me even when I lose only one pound per week?

Two brief calls to your sup buddy should be made in the morning and midday. A longer one should be made in the evening to talk about your accomplishments of that day or if you missed the mark. Do not be too hard on yourself. The key is not to give up, but to pick it up again. I tell you, it was quite a struggle for me, but I persevered. You know what? I lost the weight! When I had a setback, I picked myself up and continued. *You have to do that also!*

Your sup buddy should be very involved in this process. Make sure to discuss your answers to the weight-loss questions in this chapter with your sup buddy.

## Physician

Make sure you have talked to your physician before starting this diet and exercise plan.

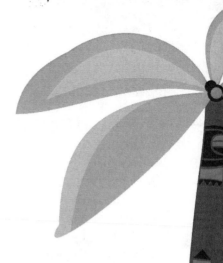

# Nutritional Knowledge

## Let's Get Familiar with Calories

It is very important that you get familiar with calories in order for you to know the calorie intake of everything you eat or drink. High-calorie items come from fat and sugar. One thing that makes a person overweight is taking in more calories than the body uses up. Make a list in your notebook of the foods and drinks you like, consume, and crave. Once your list is ready, take it to the supermarket to look up the calories per serving on the product label. Write the information in your notebook. Don't forgot to add to your list sweets (such as puddings, chocolate, pastries, and ice cream) as well as snacks (like chips, pretzels, nuts, etc.).

This self-made calorie list will get you familiar with the amount of calories per serving. See the chart in the back of the book as an aide. This knowledge will enable you to make wise decisions on how much to eat of one product or not to eat it at all. High-calorie products should be avoided completely until you have reached your desired weight. Remember, eating products high in calories will rob you of your weight loss.

At a party, you should be able to visually estimate the calories in the food and beverage items being served. Try to stay away from high-calorie foods and drinks. Parties usually offer healthy snacks like raw vegetables. If you like something other than veggies, you may have two cubes of cheese, one cracker, or a piece of meat (no sausage or salami). Think small portions. If you must have something sweet, one bite will suffice. Do not hang out at the food table—you might get tempted. Move away, take a sip of water, and pop a piece of chewing gum in your mouth. *Do not consume more than six pieces of gum a day* since chewing gum is made with sweeteners.

Likewise for beverages; know the calories per drink. At a party have one soft or hard drink only. Drink it slowly and have a glass of water next to your drink. Unsweetened tea is a better choice since it has no sugar, therefore you can have more than one. Try not to drink more than one diet soda since the artificial sweetener might still cause weight gain and the sweetener is not very healthy. Do your research on how many calories there are in a glass of soda, a coffee drink, wine, beer, etc.; these items should be included on your calorie list and excluded from your diet.

When you are able to control your food and beverage intake, you have got it! You will maintain your desired weight for the rest of your life.

> "Above all be of single aim; have a legitimate and useful purpose, and devote yourself unreservedly to it."
>
> *James Allen*

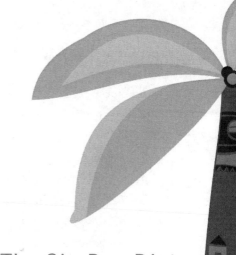

# The Six-Day Diet

Follow the diet for six days, preferably from Monday to Saturday. Sunday would be your day off. No diet and exercise. It is the day to eat in moderation some of the stuff you like. Eat every three hours; your last meal, dinner, should not be taken later than 7 p.m. Drink five to ten glasses of water a day.

## Breakfast (between 6:30 a.m.–7:30 a.m.)

An omelet made of

1/3 cup egg-white omelet or eggbeaters

Stuff with:

1 slice low or fat-free cheese

½-1 oz grilled chicken breast or cooked
    shrimps (occasionally)

1 slice tomato, avocado or bell peppers

Serve with:

1 slice whole grain bread, plain or toasted

6 oz V8 vegetable drink, plain or spicy

1 wedge fresh papaya or pineapple or apple

Once a week, you may have two organic eggs over easy or soft/hard-boiled eggs.

Beverages: water, tea or decaf coffee with fat-free half-and-half with no sugar

How to make a *healthy* omelet, using the above ingredients:

Put ½ tablespoon of virgin olive oil in a frying pan; let it heat, then add egg white or egg beater. Cover and let it cook on high to medium heat till solid. Flip over the omelet and add to one side the chicken breast or shrimps, tomato, and slice of cheese. Cover with the other half of the omelet and let it fry till light brown. Use veggies to your liking—such as tomatoes, onions, mushrooms, bell peppers, spinach, or avocado. You could lightly sauté the vegetables before stuffing the omelet. You could also make scrambled eggs; however, fry the egg white or egg substitute first on one side till light brown then scramble with the veggies, cheese, and meat. Use sea salt instead of regular salt.

## Snack (between 9:30 a.m.-10:30 a.m.)

Choose two items from this list:

½ small apple

½ banana

½ orange or a small tangerine

½ grapefruit

½ slice fresh pineapple

½ slice fresh papaya

½ slice watermelon

1 low-fat string white cheese stick

1- 6 oz yogurt, fat-free, 60–80 *cal*.

Make sure that you pick one protein item, cheese, or yogurt.

Or instead of the two snack items listed above you may choose one of the following:

2 slices Kavli *thin* whole grain plain
crisp bread,
1 wedge Laughing cow light cheese
¼ orange or mandarin
  (the Kavli thin whole grain garlic or
  pesto crisp bread is much higher
  in sodium)

a bowl of cereal with fruits
1/3 cup organic flax plus multi bran cereal
  (Nature's Path)
1/3 cup organic frozen or fresh blueberries,
  5 frozen organic cranberries,
  (the berries are high in antioxidants)
1/3 banana (if you do not like bananas,
  add 1/8 cup organic raisins
1/2 cup organic unsweetened low fat vanilla
  almond beverage

Beverages: water, tea, or decaf coffee with fat-free half-and-half, with no sugar.

Do not drink more than two cups of decaf coffee a day. Decaf coffee[1] is processed with chemicals such as methylene chloride and ethyl acetate, which could be harmful when daily three or more cups are consumed. Likewise caffeine[2] can cause or worsen several health problems when consumed. Caffeine is found in coffee beans, tea leaves, cacao seeds, and kola nuts. Caffeine stimulates the central nervous system and the cardiac muscle.

Caffeine is a drug, and it elevates blood glucose and sugar levels, as well causing us to lose calcium. It can also cause sudden severe headaches.

Teas, both green and black comes from the botanical, Camellias sinensis, which contain caffeine. However, ½ to 1/3 less than the same serving of coffee. Herbal teas are made from botanical infusions not related to Camellias sinensis and are natural caffeine free. Teas are a good Vitamin C source, however, it should also be taken in moderation, like 3 servings of preferably herbal tea per day or 1 serving of green tea and 2 servings of herbal tea, in addition to the 2 servings of decaf coffee

## Lunch (between 12 p.m.-1 p.m.)

Main course: choose one protein and one carb item

    3–4 oz grilled fish, shrimps, chicken or
        turkey breast

    1–1 ½ cup vegetables (you may steam, sauté
        or stir fry)

    ½ cup brown rice, whole grain pasta (rice 4
        days a week)

    ¼ sweet potato

side salad with ½ tablespoon of low fat
   natural dressing like Newman's Own
½ cup red kidney, pinto, navy, or
   black beans.

Dessert: choose one item
   1 piece ( 1" by 1 ½ " of dark chocolate
      65% cacao or higher, and a wedge of fruit
      (have the chocolate first then the fruit
      and then a glass of water)
   1 fruit-bar popsicle
   1/2 fiber organic power bar
   12 dried or fresh organic berries blend
      and four whole almonds
   small organic apple (organic so that the
      skin can be consumed)

Beverages: water, hot or iced tea with no sugar.
Lemon is okay to use

Once a week you may substitute your lunch main
course for a whole grain sandwich or whole grain tor-
tilla wrap with 3–4 oz.of a protein items (fish, shrimps
or white meat and 1 wedge or slice of fat free cheese) as
listed above. Use mustard but no butter or mayonnaise.

You may have it with it a side salad and ½ tablespoon of low fat natural dressing. Dessert.

## Snack (between 3 p.m.-4 p.m.)

Choose 2 items from this list
- 5–6 celery stick
- 5–6 cucumber slices
- 5–6 cherry tomatoes
- 5–6 baby carrots
- 5–6 bell pepper strips
- 1 6-oz V8, spicy or plain

Veggie Dip: choose one item, 2 tablespoons
- 2 cream cheese, fat-free topped with
  chopped up with parsley
- 2 salsa with cilantro
- 2 hummus

Beverages: water, hot or iced tea, like green tea, hibiscus flower herb tea, no sugar

If the snack does not hold you, increase the amount of veggies and have another wedge of the laughing cow light cheese.

## Dinner (between 6 p.m.-7 p.m.)

A salad made with romaine or mix spring lettuce.

Top the greens with one protein item and 3 or 4 vegetables

> 3–4 oz. grilled breast of chicken, turkey,
>> fish, canned tuna in water, cooked
>> large shrimps
>
> vegetables: cucumber, tomato, onions,
>> broccoli, cauliflowers, asparagus,
>> bean sprouts, green beans,
>> zucchini, carrots
>
> 15 almond slices or roasted soy beans
>
> ½ tablespoon ground flaxseed
>
> 2 tablespoon low fat natural dressing,
>> like Newman's Own

*(If you have the salad for lunch you may have a slice of whole grain bread or up to 5 Kavli whole grain crisp bread. You may also have ½ cup of homemade bean soup. If you have it for dinner, you should stick to the above menu without bread products and bean soup)*

Or make an entrée **without** pasta, rice, sweet potato. Choose from one protein item

> 3–4 oz grilled chicken, turkey, fish, shrimp
>
> 1–1 ½ cup vegetables

*Dessert:*

    2 cubes homemade ice-cream cubes
        (see recipe below) or
    ½ cup cold almond vanilla beverage,
        unsweetened with 1/3 cup of
        frozen blueberries

Beverages: water, tea, like green or herbal tea with no sugar. Lemon to your liking

## Hungry Late at Night?

If you are hungry before bedtime you may have one item:

    6 oz V8 vegetable juice, regular or spicy
    1 wedge Laughing cow light cheese
    ¼ cup raw or steamed vegetables

## Water

Preferably drink distilled water, five to ten glasses daily. In addition to water, as a treat, you may have sparkling water, like Syfo Or make a pitcher of cold
    —green or herbal tea, my favorite is
        Mrs. Mango's Hibiscus Flower Herb
        tea [3] without sugar; keep it cold in the

fridge. You may add lemon and/or
orange peels

—distilled water, cold, with slices of
cucumber and a mint leaf

—iced decaf coffee. Remember: only
two cups of decaf coffee a day

## Vegetables

Vitamin C[4] is also found in vegetables like broccoli, Brussels sprout, peppers, parsley and collard greens. Some of the vegetables that have anticancer properties are cabbage, broccoli, cauliflower, Brussels sprouts, radishes, soybeans, tomatoes, and garlic. Raw vegetables have the enzymes that the body need. Enzymes protect our cells, are critical to health, and are essential in the digestion and assimilation of food. Steamed or cooked vegetables destroy the enzymes[5]. Have at least one portion of uncooked veggies a day. A salad will do.

## Low-Calorie Gourmet Food

Be creative in your cooking. Use fresh herbs and spices to enhance flavor.

Use dill, lemongrass, cilantro, rosemary, ginger, etc. for salads, meat, fish, veggies. Go Mexican, Cuban, Italian,

Japanese, Thai, Hawaiian, etc; Hawaiians and Hawaiians at heart may enjoy one tablespoon of poi twice a week.

## Tips

Make sure to wash fruits and vegetables with a mild soap and a soft brush before storing in the fridge or cooking when you buy non-organic. Natural grown chicken and organic eggs, free range, are a better choice. It only costs a little bit more than regular grown. Berries, dried fruits, nuts and half and half cream should be organic.

Lightly sautéed or stirfry meat and/or veggies means a little bit of olive oil and water. (Newman's Own as an organic virgin olive oil on the market)

Use Teeccino Mocha caffeine-free herbal coffee as a treat in the evening. It is made of roasted herbs, grains, fruits and nuts. A health food store would carry it.

Just because you are now eating healthy and balanced, it does not mean that you can eat in excess. Healthy food can be high in calories. Watch calories and portions!

If you want to lose a quick pound work in the yard. Pull weeds and trim plants. Be busy for a few hours. If you do not have a yard, you could help friends with theirs.

## Do not skip meals

You *must* start your day with breakfast. Some people think that if they skip a meal, they will lose the weight faster. Not true. You must eat to keep your body sugar from dropping and keep your energy level up. Also you want to keep your body in the *fat-burning mode* by eating every three hours. Also, if you do not eat enough, your body will send a signal that it is starving and will store calories instead of burning it. Your body will burn muscle tissue. You have to eat to burn fat. *Eat less calories, not less food, and do not skip meals.*

## Plan and Prepare

*If you fail to plan, you plan to fail.* You will find this diet to be very easy to follow. Prepare your meals and snacks ahead of time. Depending on your work schedule, you might have to partly prepare your meals and snacks the night before or in the morning at breakfast time. Make sure that you pack your snacks and meal(s) for work. *Do not leave the house empty handed.* The key is to decide daily what you want to eat the next day. Write your daily meals and snack choices in your notebook and prepare. *Keep sugarless chewing gum for the moments when you crave something in-between meals.*

## Shopping

Do your shopping twice a week. Make a shopping list with the items you will need for three or four days. You can buy some frozen fish fillets in a pack if you do not mind fresh frozen fish like Pacific salmon, etc; fillets defrost fast. Also get some packs of frozen vegetables to have in the freezer, to use when you are short on time. Chicken and turkey breast can be found freshly grilled in the supermarket. *Do **not** buy or eat dark chicken or turkey meat or skin because it is higher in saturated fat thus higher in calories than white meat.*

As an aide see the shopping list in the back of the book.

## If you like sweets, don't get tempted!

Stay away from stores selling sweets like baked goods, ice cream, candy, chocolate, and coffee shops with pastries. Use the drive through if you want coffee, but remember: no sugar!

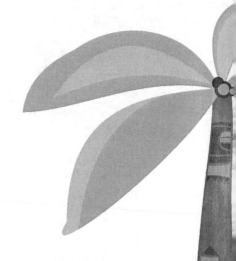

# The No and Yes foods

## No Foods:

Bacon
Bagels
Blended Coffee Drinks
Butter
Burritos
Caffeine
Chicken Pot Pies
Chicken Wings

Chips

Chocolate milk

Cookies

Corn, only if you must, occasionally

Diet bars

Donuts

Fast Food, except a side salad

French Fries

Fried Food

Fruit Juices

Hamburgers

Hot dogs, sausages, salami, or any
    other *processed meat*

Liver

Margarine

Mayo

Pastries, pies, puddings, or any other
    *baked sweet*

Potato

Processed Food

Sauces

Sodas

White bread

White rice

White pasta

White sugar

Quiches

## Be aware of calories

Pastries and French fries can have more than 600 calories per portion. Blended coffee drinks and ice-blended drinks can have more than 900 calories.

Likewise for breakfast in a restaurant; healthy choices in a restaurant don't include an omelets, bacon, cheese, home fries, or pancakes with sausages. A hamburger meal from a restaurant can easily have 700 plus calories. *Become a calorie connoisseur.*

> Remember your body uses calories as fuel to run. If you intake more than your body needs, it stores it. We can see it on our hips, waist, thighs, etc. Basically if you eat too many calories, you gain weight. If you cut calories, you lose weight.

## Yes, Limited

Almonds

Avocado

Beans, black, red, lentils, lima, no can

Butter

Brown bread

Brown rice

Brown pasta

Brown sugar

Cereal, bran or whole-grain

Cheese, low or fat-free

Chewing gum, sugarless

Coffee, decaffeinate only

Cottage Cheese, light or fat-free

Cream, organic fat-free Half- &-Half

Crisp bread, whole grain

Dark Chocolate

Diet Soda, limit to one daily

Eggs, organic

Fish: sole, orange roughy, red snapper,
  Pacific salmon, mahi-mahi, trout,
  Halibut, or tilapia

Fruits, fresh and dried

Macadamia nuts

Meat, lean

Milk, fat-free only, preferable organic

Mustard

Oatmeal, whole grain

Oil, organic extra-virgin olive oil

Popsicle, fruit bar only

Ricotta cheese, fat free

Salad Dressing, Newman's Own Light,
    natural

Salsa

Shrimps

Soy Milk, organic, low fat

Sweet Potato

Tea, green or herbal

Tuna, Albacore or Tongol

Walnuts

Yogurt, organic, fat free
    (in the 60–80 cal. range)

*Dried berries-like blueberries, raspberries and nuts—like almonds, macadamia and walnuts—are healthy to eat; however, they are high in fat. Have a small portion, like four nuts and ten berries . Remember to get organic.*

# Protein, Fiber, Fat, Salt, Sugar and the Glycemic Index

## Protein

You should have protein[1] at least three times a day. Our body structure is largely protein, and all parts of the body need protein in some way for survival. Hormones, genes, the secretion of the thyroid and pituitary gland, insulin, antibodies, enzymes, hemoglobin are protein. The heart, liver, kidneys, and eyes are made of protein. Our hair and skin are 98% protein. In order for the body to perform efficiently, it needs a continuous daily supply of protein. Protein cannot be stored in the body for long. Lack of protein weakens the muscle tone and makes us flabby. The facial muscles start to droop, and the skin begins to shrivel and wither, says Linda Clark, M.A. Prolonged protein deficiency can cause serious health problems like anemia, kidney, liver disease, low blood sugar, low blood pressure, and high cholesterol. I found that eating protein helped with my sweet cravings; it also gave me a greater feeling of fullness. Protein is necessary for weight loss, health, and vitality. If you divide your body weight in half, you will get the approximate amount of grams of protein you need daily. The general recommendation is 1 gram of protein for 2.2 pounds of body weight; however, the recommended amount of protein varies by country. In America, it is 55 grams for women and 65 grams for men. Proteins found in animal products are the complete proteins known as the amino acids. There are twenty-two of these amino acids. Other complete proteins are soybean, brewer's yeast, and wheat germ.

Interesting thing is that if one important amino acids is missing at a meal, it cannot be made up by another meal later. The drawback of vegetable protein is that it lacks B12, which can cause—when the body is depleted—nerve degeneration. Protein deficiency might not show right away; however, it creeps up behind the scenes and can eventually bring about the ailments as listed above.

Don Colbert, M.D. in his book *The Seven Pillars of Health* warns that high amounts of protein consumption since it a can put a strain on the kidneys.[3]

## Fiber

Increase fiber intake slows the absorption of fats; calories leave your body in the stool. Fiber absorbs water and retains sugar, thus slowing absorption of sugar calories by the body. Fiber comes from plant foods, fruits, and vegetables. When fiber reaches the colon, the soluble fiber is fermented by bacteria living in the colon and can be partially absorbed and digested. The insoluble fiber passes through the body with no absorption or digestion, like a sweeping broom. Soluble fiber helps to lower cholesterol and to controls blood sugar[4]. Flaxseed is a good source of fiber and so is citrus pectin that comes from the cell walls of citrus fruits. Women should have daily about 25 grams of fiber and men about 35 grams. Remember, we need fiber to lose weight.

—Soluble fiber is in fruits, oats, barley, legumes, flaxseed, and carrots.

—Insoluble fiber is in bran, wheat and rye products, the skin fruits, and vegetables.

According to Don Colbert, M.D. if a diet is low in fiber, it gives more opportunity for parasites to attach to the intestine and for toxins to enter the bloodstream [5]

## Fat

There are good and bad fats. The good fats remove excess glucose, cholesterol, and triglycerides from the bloodstream until needed. Vitamin A,D,E, and K cannot function in the body without fat. The gallbladder needs fat to work.[6]

There are four general groups of dietary fats[7]:

*Monounsaturated fats,* good fat, is found in olive oil, avocados, macadamia nuts, almonds, and flaxseed oil.

*Saturated fats* are present in animal products, red meat, pork, dark meat and skin of chicken, turkey, cold cuts, hot dogs, sausage, salami, duck, and goose. It is also found in coconut, palm oil, and **chocolate**. The body needs the benefits of small amounts of saturated fat; consume no more than 10%. Therefore, eat saturated fat products in moderation since excessive amounts will increase the risk of heart disease.

*Trans fats,* also called hydrogenated fats (bad fats), are found in margarine; shortening; processed foods like cookies, cakes, and pies; and many salad dressings. Trans fat is more damaging to your arteries than saturated fat. Olive oil and monounsaturated fats are the best choices for consumption.

Polyunsaturated fats should be consumed daily in small amounts. Excessive consumption can cause the formation of free radicals, which are associated with cancer, heart, and other diseases. Polyunsaturated fats are in pecans, walnuts, almonds, pistachios, brazil nuts and pine nuts, as well as in products like mayonnaise, corn oil, soybean oil, sunflower oil. Antioxidants slow down and neutralize the free radicals. The key is moderation. Watch your fat intake; do not clog your arteries. Do not intake more than 25 grams of fat a day.

## Oil

The three conventional methods[8] of extracting oils from nuts, grains, beans, seeds and olive are:

*the hydraulic press method*, also called cold pressed (olive oil);

*the expeller press method*, where heat is used twice;

*the solvent extraction*, in which a chemical is used to dissolve the oil. Hydrogenation is a chemical process to make fats solid, such as margarine (not a wise choice to consume).

## Salt

The scientific name for salt is sodium chloride[9]. The sodium component makes up 40 % of salt. The daily sodium dietary intake guideline is 1100 to 3300 mg.

Usually we consume four times more. Excessive sodium intake can contribute to health problems such as elevated blood pressure, headaches, fatigue, constipation etc. states William Manahan, M.D. Consuming extra salt brings more water from our intestines into the circulatory systems, thus forming more blood. Extra blood makes the heart pump faster[10]. It is not wise to consume high amounts of salt. A way to cut down on salt is by seasoning food with herbs and spices. Sea salt is a much better choice because it has potassium which can regulate the sodium by draining excess water. There are many more minerals in sea salt. Make sure to get a natural whole one. There is even one on the market with iodine. Like Redmond Real Sea Salt. Look in a health food store and check the labels.

## Sugar

Sugar belongs to the carbohydrate family. Three categories of sugar are diverse from both a chemical and nutritional point of view. *Polysaccharides* are complex sugars such as bread, pasta, potatoes, and rice. *Disaccharides* are sucrose, like table sugar, and maltose. *Monosaccharides* are found in glucose and fructose. Sugar[11] is addictive and affects our health when consumed in high amounts. Sugar should be consumed in small amounts. Likewise for artificial sweeteners. An excessive sugar intake contributes to health problems It can weaken the immune system, elevates cholesterol, leads to type 2 diabetes, speeds up the aging process, contributes to lack of energy, poor concentration and memory, and it affects our behaviors and moods. It also makes us fat. Excess sugar (empty calories) robs stored vitamins and minerals from the body. Likewise for artificial sweeteners. Raw brown natural sugar is a better choice than white sugar and should be consumed in small amounts. Sugar is hidden in food products like cereal, yogurts, ketchup, soups, medication, etc. Generally our sugar consumption should not be more than 10% of our total caloric intake, however, it should be minimal when following a weight loss diet.

(The two levels of chemicals—serotonin, found in sugary and starchy food, and dopamine,[12] found in chocolate—are raised when we eat those foods which boost our comfort level).

## Glycemic Index

This system ranks food rich in carbohydrates based on their effect on the glycemia, in other words their ability to raise or lower blood sugar levels following consumption. A low glycemic index of 50 represents carbohydrates that are absorbed slowly, releasing glucose gradually into the bloodstream while a high glycemic index of 100 or higher indicates a rapid absorption producing high glycemic spikes. A sudden spike in glycemia stimulates the release of insulin, which stores glucose in cells. The body wants more sugars because of the fall of the blood glucose levels, consequently stimulating the desire to eat. The high glycemic index (GI foods) includes sweets, biscuits, potato, white bread, rice, and sugary drinks.

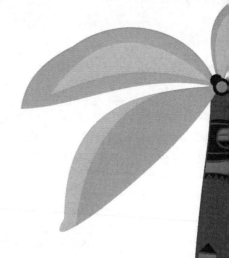

# Toxins & Nutrients

## Milk

Antibiotics are usually used to treat diary cows for infections. Cows are fed with grains that have pesticides, industrial waste, etc. These toxins concentrate in the fatty tissue of the animals and in the diary products. Whole milk and whole milk products, like butter, cheese, and ice cream, have high pesticide residue[13]. Use low fat and skim milk and low or fat free milk products. Preferably use organic milk and milk products.

## MSG

Monosodium glutamate[14] is a sodium salt, an ingredient in processed food that enhances the taste to stimulate your appetite. MSG is found in ice creams, soy sauce, dry milk powder, salad dressings, and processed meats as well as processed foods in restaurants (like fried chicken, sausage, etc.) MSG can cause obesity and harm the brain neurons, stated Don Colbert, M.D. Furthermore, by consuming MSG the blood sugar drops and makes you hungry. MSG can be labeled under different names like hydrolyzed vegetable protein, yeast extract, soy protein isolate, artificial flavors, etc.

## Processed food

Processed food usually contains chemicals like preservatives to prolong shelf life, flavoring, coloring, bleaching agents, etc. The food is usually made with lots of calories and little nutrition. Eating processed food can make you deficient in proper nutrients. Most degenerative diseases such as, diabetes, arthritis, heart decease and cancer are usually associated with nutritional deficiencies[15], states Don Colbert, M.D.

For the sake of good health, limit your consumption.

## Red meat

Red meat has a higher concentration of toxins than other foods. The animal stores the toxins (like pesticides, antibiotics, and hormones) in its fat[16]. When you consume that good tasting fat (for some people), you put the same toxins in your body. Your liver then has to process and eliminate the toxins. If it is too much for the liver to eliminate it gets stored in your fatty tissue. Eat lean meat and limit your intake and portion. Likewise for chicken. Turkey breast is the leanest meat with less toxins and animal fat. Organic, free-range, or grass-fed meats are better choices.

## Toxins

We are exposed to toxins everywhere. In the air, water, buildings, food, and chemicals, as well as in our body. Our bodies battle toxins everyday and work hard to break down and eliminate the toxins. Toxins create a health risk, and several chemicals cause cancer. When someone lights up a cigarette, that person releases over 2,000 chemicals in that smoke. Secondhand smoke[17] is even more harmful because of the hazardous chemicals released from the lighted end. The smoke produces free radicals and can cause lung cancer. One in every five deaths is related to smoking. Every time a smoker puffs on a cigarette[18] or cigar he plants a seed for lung cancer states Don Colbert, M.D. He also states that studies have shown that smokers should **not** take beta carotene as a supplement because it increases the instance of lung cancer in smokers.

## Free radicals

Free radicals[19] damage and destruct our cells. They come from normal metabolism and production of energy in our bodies. Free radicals are created by excessive intake of certain foods like sugar, fried foods, processed foods, polyunsaturated fats found in salad dressings, cooking oils, sauces, etc. Free radicals are also found in hydrogenated fats, diseases like cancer, asthma, coronary heart disease, colds, flu, etc. Even excessive exercise can create free radicals. The liver[20], our filter, is busy all day long filtering our blood to cleanse and detox it before the blood goes back into circulation. Toxins enter our body through food, water, parasites, air, yeast and bacteria growth in the small intestines. In the detoxification process of the toxins can produce free radicals. Antioxidants protects us from free radicals.

## Antioxidants

An Antioxidant[21] is a vitamin, a mineral, an enzyme, a phyto nutrient[22] or a food. They have the ability to neutralize free radicals. Antioxidants are also produced by our bodies. Green tea is a powerful antioxidant and so are red, blue, purple, green, and yellow fruits and vegetables, like berries, tomato. Spinach, carrots, apples, and tangerines.

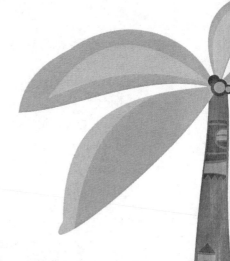

# Sunday Diet & Eating Out

It is Sunday, your day off the diet and exercise. You should eat in moderation. Plan your day and menu. Look up your calorie allowance. It is important that you count calories. Stay away from calorie-rich food. Following are suggestions of what you may have on this day.

## Breakfast:

1 slice bacon, if you must,
    or 1 vegetable breakfast patty

2 eggs over easy, scrambled, or hard-boiled

Choose one item
  1 slice whole grain bread
  ½ whole grain muffin
  1 whole grain waffle
  ½ bran muffin, low fat
  8 oz rice protein shake

  Protein Shake:
2 scoops of rice protein, ¼ cup of frozen berries, ½ tablespoon of flaxseed oil, and ½ tablespoon of ground flaxseed; you may use banana or papaya instead of the berries. Blend with ice until semi thick. Add a pinch of salt.)

  or

  Fast Food Restaurant:
Choose items that are low cal. If you like to know the calorie content of fast food before you pick it up or dine, I recommend you purchase a food counter guide, one that features the restaurants in the book. Get a complete guide that also lists the protein, carbohydrates, fat, and fiber per food or drink item.

  When ordering ask to omit or to put on the side fattening items. For instance if you order the Asian

Sesame Chicken Salad from Panera Bread ask for the dressing on the side, no wontons. Ask for a piece (half of a ¼ ) of whole grain baguette instead of the white.

There you are—a low calorie, nutritious meal. Remember, no more than 2 tablespoons of salad dressing and no butter on the baguette. When choosing a soup, look for the ones that are not made with cream, potato, pasta, rice or cheese.

or

Homemade breakfast quiche, *see recipe*
   ½ a fruit
   1 packet oatmeal, instant "low-sugar"

Beverages: water, decaf coffee with fat-free half-and-half cream, green tea or iced tea, no Sugar.

## Lunch

Choose one item
   1 slice cheese pizza
   homemade sirloin hamburger, or vegetable
      patty on whole wheat "light" bun
   ½ whole-wheat pita bread stuffed with
      meat or fish and veggies to your liking

*Dessert:* Choose one item
½ cup plain ice cream, fat-free
½ cup sherbet, low or fat-free
¼ slice pie
*Remember, it is not good for you but if you must stick to the suggested portion.*

## Dinner

You may have red lean meat if you like. Choose one meat item.

> 3–4oz grilled top round steak, cube steak
>   sirloin chop steak, lean pork.
> 1–1 ½ cups vegetables
> 1 side salad with 1/2 tablespoon of low fat
>   natural dressing. *Preferably do not eat
>   rice, sweet potato, pasta with this meal;
>   but if you must have it, just have ½ a cup
>   or ¼ sweet potato. It is better to have it
>   for lunch.*

> *Dessert*: choose one item
>   ½ slice pineapple, papaya, watermelon
>   ½ apple, pear, orange

## Eating Out

Eat only *half* of what you ordered. Try to stay away from fried foods; pastas; rich, creamy, or buttery sauces; pastries; and ice cream. Have a small portion of sherbet or a piece of fruit. Order low-calorie food and eat only half of it. Ask right away for a to-go box so that you can put half away as soon as the food arrives. Take dressings and sauces on the side. Sushi is okay, but half portions only.

## Alcohol

If you drink alcohol, you may have it once a week only, preferably on the day that your are off the diet.

Your options are:

> ½ glass of wine or non-alcoholic wine
>
> 1 glass or small bottle of light beer or
>
>     non-alcoholic beer.

Stay away from mixed drinks with or without multiple alcohol and fruit juices, including the virgin ones.

## One Bite of One Item—Sundays Only

You may have one bite of anything on your "no" list, like baked potato, cake, French fries, etc. *One item only* if somebody else in your company is eating that. If one bite is going to tempt you to take more than one, you should *not* take a bite. This is only for strong dieters.

## Substitute

You may substitute certain items with the same nutritional values for others; however, make sure that they have more or less the same calories per serving. Do not substitute protein for non-protein food items. You must have protein everyday.

*Do not substitute the "no" items for "yes" items. The no items will sabotage your weight loss; most of them are not nutritious and not good for your health.*

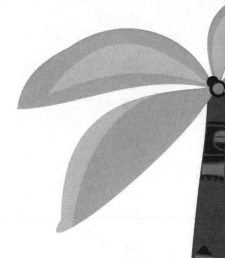

# Recipes

## Ice cream cubes

Mix one pint of fat-free milk and two teaspoons each of almond and vanilla extract; add some freshly grated ginger to taste and two teaspoons of brown raw sugar, honey, or maple syrup. After you mix the elements, pour in an ice tray and freeze.

## Pickled cucumber

Make pickled cucumber. Mix apple cider vinegar (diluted), a pinch of salt, and brown sugar to taste. Slice cucumber, no skin or seeds, add salt, then put in a jar. If you wish, you may add some sliced onions and/or a whole, fresh green pepper. Let stand for about two hours, then put in the fridge

## Homemade Breakfast Quiche

Take ½ of a whole wheat or grain muffin; pour egg white in the bun, allowing it to soak into the muffin. Add soft fat-free cheese, then add toppings to your liking—such as cut up pieces of grilled chicken breast, turkey breast, or poached fish and some veggies. Then top with some more egg white. Put on a lightly buttered tray (grease it with butter or olive oil) then place in the toaster oven for about 7 to 10 minutes on 350 degrees. Feel free to add salt and spices to taste. You may also lightly sauté the veggies before adding them to the muffin.

## Oven roasted tomatoes

Cut two vine grape tomatoes in slices and place in a casserole dish. Add salt and white or black pepper to taste, cut up two fresh basil leaves, mix with extra virgin olive oil, and put in a toaster oven for 20–30 minutes on 350 degrees. Sprinkle with a tablespoon of parmesan grated cheese and freshly cut up parsley when done

## Okra Soup

Make a broth. Bring to boil 16 oz of distilled water then add 1 diced tomato and ½ an onion and add sea salt and black pepper to taste. Let boil for 10 minutes. Slice up 4 okras and 12 spinach leaves and add to the bouillon. Boil for another 15 minutes until ready. You may add some diced grilled chicken or fish to the soup.

## Fish Soup

Bring to boil 16 oz. of distilled water and make a broth; add some celery. Take 1 or 2 fillets of fish—like tilapia or orange roughy—sprinkle lightly with organic lemon pepper spice, then dice the fillets and add to the bouillon. Cook for 15 minutes. You may add some frozen small peas or other veggies to the soup.

## Chicken Fillets

Lightly sprinkle both sides of two chicken breast thin fillets with Montreal steak and rosemary spices. Do not add salt since the Montreal steak spice has salt in the mix. Moisten fillets with a touch of virgin olive oil. Likewise add 3–4 drops of virgin olive oil on the toaster oven tray before placing in the toaster oven. Grill for ten to fifteen minutes, depending on the thickness of the fillets, at 375 degrees.

## Saute Chicken

Cut up or slice a 2 lbs of natural chicken breast fillets, sprinkle with Montreal steak spices, ½ tablespoon of sea salt, 1 tablespoon of rosemary spice and 1 tablespoon of olive oil.

Dice both an onion, garlic and a tomato, add 2 cups of filtered water. When the water boils add the marinated chicken. Cook on high for 30 minutes then 10 minutes on high to medium heat. This amount will last you for at least three days. Store the chicken breast in a container in the fridge and use as needed. Use different spices to make different flavored chicken breast. Go Italian, Mexican, Thai etc. Be creative.

Moana would have added to the above seasoning 2 tablespoons of Newman's Own teriyaki marinade, 1 tablespoon of lemon grass leaves, and 1/4 cup of coconut milk, for the last 10 minutes of cooking.

(Rinse your chicken prior to cooking, prepare a bowl of water add 1 tablespoon of vinegar. Remove chicken breast from the packet and place in the bowl. Let sit for 2 minutes, drain then cut up the breast)

## Moana's Lilikoi Fish (passion fruit)

Cut up 1 or 2 fillets of fish (like snapper, tilapia, or orange roughy) and season with salt and black pepper. Bring to boil ½ -1 cup of water, add ¼ sliced onion.

Mix one-tablespoon raw brown sugar with 1/8 cup of lilikoi pulp. Add the fish pieces and lilokoi mix. Cook for about five minutes then add 1/8 diced fresh, sweet pineapple. Cook for another 8–10 minutes.

## Moana's Coconut Cabbage

Bring to boil ¾ cup of water; add 1 tablespoon of fresh or powder onion, garlic and raw brown sugar. Add two cups of cabbage. Salt to taste and add ½ teaspoon of raw brown sugar. Boil for about 10 minutes till cabbage is semi tender, then add 1/8 cup coconut milk, and stir. Cook for another minute. Top with one crushed or chopped macadamia nut. (Do not throw away any water/juice that is left from cooking the cabbage. It is delicious and is rich in nutrients; enjoy it!)

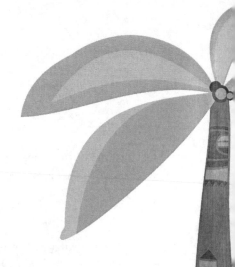

# Daily Calorie Allowance

### Calories: Women—weekdays

1250–1400 calories per day during the week

### Calories: Women—Sundays

1400–1600 calories on this day.

### Calories: Men—Weekdays

1550–1700 calories per day during the week

## Calories: Men—Sundays

1700 -1900 calories on this day.

## Men

The portions in this book are based on women. Men may have 10%-15% more.

## Check Your Weight

On Sunday morning get on the scale and record your new weight in your notebook. On Monday morning get on the scale and record your starting weight. Weigh yourself only twice a week. Stay away from the scale during the week. Put it away so that you do not see it. *The scale is not your friend during the week.*

## Take a Picture

Record your success! A neat thing to do is to take a picture every month, so that you can see your weight loss and your new look. (Do not forget to stick your tongue out and make a face) A picture paints a thousand words! Paste it in your journal.

## Setbacks

Setbacks occur when you have not followed your diet but instead ate more than you were supposed to. You might have them from time to time. Keep your chin up and start again with the diet. Look back to see where you failed. Was it emotions, or were you tempted because it tasted so good ? Learn from your setbacks and try to do it differently the next time when you are tempted.

## Sleep

Thank God for giving us sleep to be able to function!

Try to go to bed no later than 10:30 p.m.; your systems need adequate sleep. Your body needs it to repair and rejuvenate itself. Cells are also being replaced. Remember the old saying, "Early to bed, early to rise, makes a man healthy, wealthy, and wise." Sleep is important to renew our cells, gain knowledge, and to be able to function properly, etc. It is said that sleep is more important to life than food. *You actually lose weight when you sleep*. Furthermore, not enough of sleep leads to an increased appetite. I know it first hand. I was an eating zombie for years.

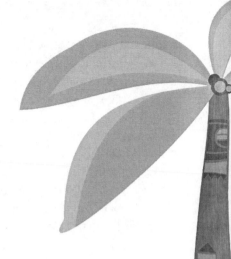

# Supplements &
# Maintenance

## Supplements

Talk to your doctor regarding the supplements you should take. A nutritionist at a health-food store will be able to assist you with your selection. In Dr. Don Colbert's book *The Seven Pillars of Health* is a chapter on Supplements[1] and how to pick the right ones that might be of help to you.

Omega 3 is beneficial for the cardiovascular system, the eyes and our over all health. It can lower triglycerides and can burn stored fat easily. The body does not make Omega 3, we have to get it from eating fish products, like salmon, fish oils and flaxseed products.

Lecithin[2] supplement is effective to lower cholesterol levels. Lecithin is made from soybeans. It also helps to evenly distribute body weight. Lecithin works slowly but well.

The multi vitamin and mineral supplement that I have been taking for at least 20 years is called Bogdana Nutritional Formula. It comes in liquid form and has more than 150 nutrients in the product.

## Detoxification

There are several products on the market. Speak to a nutritionist at a health-food store if you wish to detoxify before starting a diet. A nutritionist can recommend a natural product.

## Maintenance

Once you have lost the weight, you will have to maintain it. Stick to your basic menus and portions. Keep the calorie knowledge of a product in mind. Keep on exercising. If you failed eating right for a day or two, start again. Keep the journey going.

You may have more calories per day; however, women should not exceed 1700–1900 per day and men should not exceed 2500–2900. Stay away from fried and fatty foods. Remember: occasionally you may have a bite of that calorie-rich food. It tastes good but it is bad for your heart and arteries. Likewise for sweets like cookies, cakes, pies and ice cream. If you look at a serving of fried chicken or fish with French fries, a roll, and coleslaw, you should close your eyes and picture the hundreds of calories that are jumping up and down from the plate. Say, "*No,* that is not for me. I am not crazy to eat that. I know that if I do, I will be at least a pound heavier tomorrow and a step closer to my grave. I choose to eat low cal, low fat, low sugar, low carb foods that do taste good. I will be healthy and feel good." *Remember: you are the Calorie and healthy choice Connoisseur.*

Try not to eat carbohydrates like bread, rice, potatoes, and pasta after 4 p.m. Watch your portions. If you are eating in a restaurant, skip the butter on the bread. Do not go overboard with rolls (with or without garlic butter), cheese sticks, muffins or pizza. Continue to stay away from white products such as bread, pasta, and rice that have no nutritional values, only calories. You may have a portion occasionally, if you must. Also stay away from high-calorie desserts. If you are tempted sometimes by sweets like cakes, pies or pastries, have a small portion or run. Stay in control. With one glance at a food dish or dessert, you should be able to convert it to calories. If it is high in calories, stay away and wave to it. Calories creep up! Do not jeopardize your accomplishment. You may eat all day if you like to but choose low calories, healthy food and drinks. Do not go over your daily calorie allowance, and by all means do your exercises.

> "A man has to learn that he cannot command things, but that he can command himself; that he cannot coerce the wills of others, but that he can mold and master his own will: and things serve him who serves Truth; people seek guidance of him who is master of himself."
>
> *James Allen*

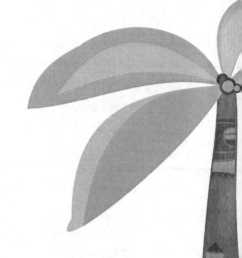

# Daily Motivation and Affirmations

Say aloud each affirmation twice. Write them on an index card. Keep the card handy so that you can pull it out and read it at least twice in the morning and in the afternoon, or anytime you need encouragement.

*Today, I am going to continue to lose weight*
*Today, I am going to continue to eat healthy*
*Today, I am going to continue to cut portions*

*Today, I am going to continue to control*
*my food intake*
*Today, I am going to continue to count calories*
*Today, I am going to continue to follow*
*this simple and easy diet*
*Today, I am going to continue my new way*
*of eating*
*Today, I am going to continue to do physical*
*exercises*
*Today, I am going to contact my buddy*
*for support*
*Today, I am going to continue to read*
*the Scriptures*
*Today, I am going to ask God to strengthen me*
*Today, I am going to succeed in being successful*
*Today, I am going to keep on working to look*
*good and be healthy*
*Today, I am going to continue my new lifestyle*

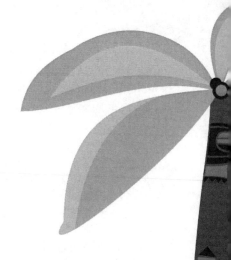

# Bible Verses, Praise Songs, and Hymns

## Bible Verses

After reading your Bible and meditating on the Bible verses, pick one or two for the week and write it on your index card. Read it often so that you can memorize the verses. The following week pick another verse and memorize it. Quote a Bible verse when you get tempted. These Bible verses become your spiritual weapon when you get tempted. Call out to the Lord as much as you need Him to get you through the day. Say, "God, I need you now, help me!" Lean on Him.

Here are a few verses that you can start with:

> "Listen to counsel and receive instruction, that you may be wise in your latter days. There are many plans in a man's heart, Nevertheless the Lord's counsel, that will stand" (Proverbs 19:20, 21).

> "For I know the thoughts that I think toward you, says the Lord, thoughts of peace and not evil, to give you a future and a hope. Then you will call upon Me and go and pray to Me, and I will listen to you" (Jeremiah 29:11, 12).

> "Through the Lord's mercies we are not consumed, Because His compassion fail not. They are new every morning, Great is Your faithfulness" (Lamentations 3:22–23).

> "Therefore, I tell you, whatever you ask in prayer, believe that you have received it and it will be yours" (Marks 11:24).

> "But each one is tempted when he draws away by his own desires and enticed" (James 1:14).

"Blessed is the man who endures temptation; for when he has been approved, he will receive the crown of life which the Lord has promised to those who love Him" (James 1:12).

"Whoever has no rule over his own spirit is like a city broken down, without walls" (Proverbs 25:28).

"The Lord is my strength and my shield; My heart trusted in Him, and I am helped; Therefore my heart greatly rejoices, and with my song I will praise Him" (Psalm 28:7).

"If you love me keep my commandments" (John 14:15).

"Yet in all things we are more than conquerors through Him who loved us" (Romans 8:37).

"Therefore do not let sin reign in your mortal body, that you should obey it in its lusts" (Romans 6:12).

"For I consider that the sufferings of this present time are not worthy to be compared with the glory which shall be revealed in us" (Romans 8:18).

"I beseech you therefore brethren, by the mercies of God, that your present bodies a living sacrifice, holy, acceptable to God, which is your reasonable service" (Romans 12:1).

"And do not be conformed to this world, but be transformed by the renewing of your mind, that you may prove what is that good and acceptable and perfect will of God" (Romans 12:2).

"Therefore submit to God, Resist the devil and he will flee from you" (James 4:7).

"I can do all things through Christ who strengthens me" (Philippians 4:13).

"Or do you not know that your body is the temple of the Holy Spirit who is in you, whom you have from God, and you are not your own" (1 Corinthians 6:19).

"Serve the Lord with gladness; Come before His presence with singing" (Psalm 100:2).

*In addition to reading your Bible, worship the Lord by singing songs and hymns to Him. There are so many to choose from.*

# Take My Life

*Scott Underwood*

Holiness, holiness is what I long for
Holiness is what I need
Holiness, holiness is what You want from me.

Faithfulness, faithfulness is what I long for
Faithfulness is what I need
Faithfulness, faithfulness is what You want from me

Chorus:
So Take my heart and form it
Take my mind ; transform it
Take my will; conform it
To Yours, To Yours, oh Lord

## As The Deer, Psalm 42:1

*Martin J. Nystrom*

As the deer panteth for the water
So my soul longeth after Thee
You alone are my heart's desire
And I long to worship thee

Chorus
You alone are my strength, my shield
To you alone may my spirit yield
You alone are my heart's desire
And I long to worship Thee

## Great is Thy Faithfulness

*Thomas Chisholm & William Runyan*

Great is Thy faithfulness, O God My Father
There is no shadow of turning with Thee
Thou changest not, Thy compassions they fail not
As Thou hast been thou forever wilt be

Great is Thy faithfulness,
Great is thy faithfulness
Morning by morning new mercies I see
All I have needed Thy hand hath provided
Great is Thy faithfulness Lord unto me

## How Great Thou Art

*Stuart K. Hine*

O Lord my God, When I in awesome wonder,
Consider all the worlds Thy Hands have made;
I see the stars, I hear the rolling thunder,
Thy power throughout the universe displayed.

Chorus
Then sings my soul, My Savior God, to Thee,
How great Thou art, How great Thou art.
Then sings my soul, My Savior God, to Thee,
How great Thou art, How great Thou art!

When Christ shall come, with shout of acclamation,
And take me home, what joy shall fill my heart.
Then I shall bow, in humble adoration,
And then proclaim: "My God, how great Thou art!"

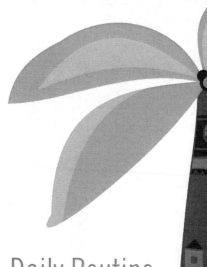

# Daily Routine

1. Start with prayer. Say good morning to God. Thank Him for the strength He gave you yesterday and ask Him for His help again to resist the temptations that may come your way today as well as strength to stay focus and stick to your weight-loss program.

2. Read your Bible and meditate on the Bible verses.

3. Ten minutes of stretching or ballet exercises and light weight lifting (5 pounds); Heavy weight lifting should be done every other day.

4. Fix and eat breakfast.

5. Pack your food.

6. Get ready for work, if you do.

7. Call your buddy.

8. Get on the road if you're going to work.

9. Have a snack at about 10 a.m.

10. Lunch between 12:30 p.m. and 1 p.m.

11. After lunch make a quick call to your buddy.

12. Afternoon snack around 3 p.m.

13. Get on the road to head home.

14. Dinner between 6 p.m.-7 p.m.

15. Exercise

16. Plan your menus and snacks for the next day.

17. Leisure time and call your buddy

18. Bed time

19. Prayer—If you did not stick to your diet, confess where you went wrong, ask the Lord to show you the way to better deal with it, and thank Him for the day. If you did, thank the Lord for the strength and guidance.

| Day | Date | Weight | | Day | Date | Weight |
|-----|------|--------|--|-----|------|--------|
| Mon | | | | Mon | | |
| Sun | | | | Sun | | |
| Loss | | | | Loss | | |

| Day | Date | Weight | | Day | Date | Weight |
|-----|------|--------|--|-----|------|--------|
| Mon | | | | Mon | | |
| Sun | | | | Sun | | |
| Loss | | | | Loss | | |

| Day | Date | Weight | | Day | Date | Weight |
|-----|------|--------|--|-----|------|--------|
| Mon | | | | Mon | | |
| Sun | | | | Sun | | |
| Loss | | | | Loss | | |

| Day | Date | Weight | | Day | Date | Weight |
|-----|------|--------|--|-----|------|--------|
| Mon | | | | Mon | | |
| Sun | | | | Sun | | |
| Loss | | | | Loss | | |

| Day | Date | Weight | | Day | Date | Weight |
|-----|------|--------|--|-----|------|--------|
| Mon | | | | Mon | | |
| Sun | | | | Sun | | |
| Loss | | | | Loss | | |

Calories

| Product | Calories | Serving Size | Fat grams | Carbs grams | Protein grams | Fiber grams |
|---|---|---|---|---|---|---|
| Laughing Cow Light Cheese | 35 | wedge | 2 | 1 | 2.5 | 0 |
| Fat Free Yogurt | 70 | 4 oz | 0 | 12 | 4.5 | 0 |
| Chicken grilled | 120 | 3 oz | 11 | 1 | 16 | 0 |
| Fat Free Half & Half Cream | 20 | 2 tbsp | 0 | 3 | 1 | 0 |
| Liquid Egg Whites | 30 | 1/4 cup | 0 | 1 | 6 | 0 |
| V8, vegetable juice | 30 | 5.5 can | 0 | 7 | 1 | 1 |
| Brown Rice cooked | 218 | 1 cup | 1 | 46 | 5 | 4 |
| Pasta whole wheat, cooked | 174 | 1 cup | 1 | 37 | 7 | 6 |
| Sweet potato, baked | 185 | 1 large | 0 | 44 | 3 | 5 |
| Snapper, raw | 218 | 1 fillet | 2 | 0 | 45 | 0 |
| Orange Roughy, raw | 59 | 3 oz | 0 | 0 | 12 | 0 |
| Tuna in water, can | 150 | 6 oz | 2.5 | 0 | 32 | 0 |
| Crispbread light rye | 30 | 1 slice | 0 | 7 | 1 | 1.5 |
| Whole grain | 80-110 | 1 slice | 1 | 15 | 3 | 2 |
| Pumpernickel | 65-100 | 1 slice | 1 | 12 | 2 | 2 |
| Black beans, cooked | 250 | 1 cup | 1 | 41 | 15 | 15 |
| Lentils, cooked | 230 | 1 cup | 1 | 40 | 18 | 16 |
| Papaya, fresh | 38 | 1/2 slice | 0 | 7 | 0.5 | 1.5 |
| Pineapple, fresh | 20 | 1/2 slice | | | | |
| Avocado | 141 | 1/2 cup, cubes | 10 | 6 | 1.5 | 6 |
| Banana | 70 | 1/2 cup, cubes | 0 | 17 | 1 | 2 |
| Grapefruit | 53 | 1/2 large | 0 | 13 | 1 | 2 |
| Orange | 32 | 1/2 | 0 | 8 | 0.5 | 1.5 |

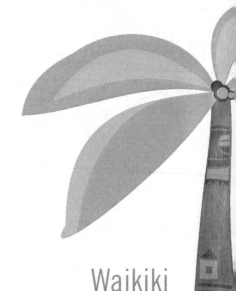

# Waikiki

## Captain Cook and the Hawaiian Royalty

As promised, there sat Moana[1], the beautiful Hawaiian woman dressed in a colorful mumuu, beneath the banyan tree under a gorgeous blue sky; framed by the dark turquoise water of the sea at midday Moana was surrounded by seven tourists visiting from California and Florida. Some were sitting on bamboo beach mats while the others sat on a bench. A Japanese couple approached and pulled up two chairs. All listened to Moana's stories of Captain Cook and the Hawaiian royal family.

Captain James Cook discovered the Hawaiian island Kauai in 1778. In January of 1779, the two ships, the *Discovery* and the *Resolution*, were anchored in Kealakekua Bay of the island of Hawaii, also called the Big Island, near the village of Kekua and Kaawaloa. Captain Cook named the Hawaiian Islands the Sandwich Islands. Captain Cook and Captain Clerke were received by the royal priests and natives in awe and with great honors. They were worshipped like a superior being when they went ashore. The priests were identifying captain Cook as their harvest god called "Lono." At that time the Hawaiians had many gods that they worshipped. The captains and some of the other officers were invited to a ceremonial feast, luau, where the natives in a processional walk carried a roasted pig, breadfruit, vegetables, and poi. The priests performed chants that ended with the word Lono. The faces, heads, shoulders, and hands of the guests were rubbed with chewed coconut, and they were fed the food by hand.

For the arrival of the great ruler Kalaniopuu of the Island of Hawaii, a kapu, a sacred law, had been ordered, and the natives were not allowed to venture out of their houses although a few officers of the two ships were trying to persuade some of the natives to trade their goods for vegetables, fruits, and meat since they were running short of food on the ships; however, the natives were fearful of their sacred law.

"Upon his arrival the ruler Kalaniopuu made an informal visit to the *Resolution* before going ashore. A formal exchange of courtesies took place the next day. The captains Cook and Clerke became friends with the ruler.

In February of 1779, Captain Cook set sail to the North, hoping to find a more protected anchorage for his ships, however, the weather got bad with strong gale force winds. Fortunately, the ships were able to ride out the storm, although, the head of the foremast of the *Resolution* was broken and needed to be repaired.

The captains decided to go back to Kealakekua Bay, and when they got there they found the villages under a second kapu since Kalaniopuu had gone away. Things came back to normal when the ruler returned and lifted the kapu. The bay natives in their canoes started to barter their food for iron and the women were offering their services. Even though the exchange of goods took place peacefully, the bay natives would steal anything they saw on the deck or on the outside of the ships. Captain Cook was puzzled by their goodwill and behavior. He wondered how their behavior could change with no apparent reason and how their curiosity could turn into an uproar of near violence like in Kauai. He also wondered about the natives' adoration that so easily turned into calculated theft in Kealakekua Bay?

He realized that it must have been equally difficult for the natives to understand the intentions of white men.

Things seemed normal. But what was normal? You never knew what the mood of the natives would be. Captain Cook was still their "Lono," their harvest god, but who were the crew members considered to be and was Captain Cook really Lono?

Captain Cook came up with a plan to invite the ruler Kalaniopuu to the *Resolution*, planning to keep him hostage so that the theft problem by the natives would cease. He also wanted the cutter of the *Resolution* back. The ruler was feared and respected by the natives and was thereby able to control them. In order to execute his plan Captain Cook went ashore to go meet with Kalaniopuu, however he did not make it very far. The Captain was held up by a group of people who had a mood shift that turned ugly when they saw Captain Cook and his marine entourage.

It became a dangerous situation. Warriors started to throw stones at the marines at the water's edge. Captain Cook was attacked with a stone and an iron spike. The Captain fired the first barrel of his musket, then raised his hand to order his marines to fire. The warriors took the signal as an affirmation for war. Captain Cook was stabbed in the back of his neck by the warriors. He fell face down and was clubbed to death.

The warriors had attacked ferociously. The body of the Captain was on the beach. It was impossible for the crew to try to take the body away. The ships were forced to turn around. The next morning the blowing of the conch shell horns signaled the arrival of more warriors. At night two natives approached the ships with a bundle containing parts of Captain Cook's body. The rest of his body was in possession of the ruler and other chiefs to perform a religious ceremony for "Lono.." Captain Clerke wanted all of Captain Cook's remains and ordered to open fire. The ruler's nephew, Kamehameha, was injured in the attack. The sailors had set the village on fire.

Twenty natives eventually walked with white flags and peace offerings, but the sailors kept on firing at them, demanding the rest of the body of the Captain. Later a chief handed over the last remains and a few of his belongings. A kapu was put on the bay to perform a naval burial. Cannons were fired in salute, and Captain Cook's bones were let down into the water, his final resting place.

The ruler, Kalaniopuu died in 1782, and his bones were placed in the royal burial house, Hale o Keawe at Honaunau. (However, in 1829 Queen Kaahumanu went to Hale o Keawe where she took the bones of the ancient chiefs and had them reburied with a Christian service.) You can visit this site at the National Historical Park *Puuhonua o Honaunau* in Kona on the Big Island.

The most powerful chief on Maui was Kahekili, who was raised as a warrior who roasted his enemies.

When he took over Oahu, he killed and sacrificed his foster son to the war god and cruelly tortured most of Oahu's chiefs to death. He had half of his body, from head to toe, tattooed in black to remind him of the thunder god.

Kamehameha ruled on the island of Hawaii, and with the help of Isaac Davis and John Young and the ship *The Fair American*, he launched an attack on Maui in 1790 and defeated the army. Because of trouble on Hawaii, the Big Island, Kamehameha had to return home.

Kahekili of Oahu, his half-brother, Kaeokulani of Kauai, a group of men and some trained warriors set sail for the island of Hawaii to harass Kamehameha. The bloody battle was fought with foreign gunners. Kahekili gave up the battle early and returned to Oahu where he met an English merchant captain William Brown in the harbor of Honolulu. Kahekili made an agreement with him to help fight Kamehameha and in return he was given the use of the harbor. He became involved in island affairs.

Kamehameha was undefeatable. In 1794, he met Captain George Vancouver who had returned as captain of the Discovery. Kamehameha made an agreement with the Captain to cede Hawaii to Britain and in return he expected an armed vessel and gifts. Captain Vancouver was a good man and had the well being of the natives at heart. He also tried to bring Kahekili and Kamehameha together to work out their differences, to make peace. His attempts were in vain. Kahekili died in Waikiki in 1794.

After Kamehameha had captured Maui and Molokai in 1795, he proceeded to Oahu by taking his fleet around the west coast between Waialae and Waikiki.

The battle was fought in the Nuuana valley. Kamehameha was fearless.

He eventually captured each island, and by 1810 he gained control of Kauai and Niihau by coming to an agreement with the chieftains. For uniting all the eight islands, he earned the title Kamehameha the Great. He was a shrewd and smart businessman-King. He died in 1819. His son Liholiho took over the reign and was named Kamehameha II.

The first whaling ships came to Hawaii, hunting whales in the island waters in 1819. The ports of Honolulu (Oahu) and Lahaina (Maui) had hundreds of ships. Buying and selling prices were at an all time high.

King Liholiho, was pressured to do away with the kapus by his mother and by Kaahumanu, the favorite wife of his father's twenty-one wives. He abolished the kapu system by breaking it to eat a meal with the female chiefs. The natives were shocked and expected their gods to punish them. At the end of his life, he took a trip to England with one of his five wives to see King George IV to discuss the British Hawaiian affairs. He and his wife fell ill and died. His brother, who was only nine years old, was proclaimed Kamehameha III. Queen Kaahumanu ruled the islands in his place.

The first Christians—Calvinist—missionaries from Massachusetts arrived in April 1820 aboard the ship *Thaddeus*. The missionaries could not go ashore until King Liholiho gave his permission, however, they were allowed a day of sightseeing Honolulu with its taro gardens, fish ponds and grass huts Their leader was Reverend Hiram Bingham. The missionaries wrote the Hawaiian alphabet, translated the Bible, and started the first schools. The natives understood that their old gods had abdicated in favor of One God, three persons. God the Father, God the Son, God the Holy Spirit. The missionaries explained to the natives that God is love and just. God cannot see nor can He accept sin. He tells us that the wages of sin is death. We all have sinned and fall short of His glory and no matter what amount of good deeds we do, we cannot be perfect and cannot have a 100% score. Therefore, the sin problem had to be dealt with before we may receive the gift of eternal life. Holy blood had to be shed to cleanse us. Because God's love for us, He sent His Son to dwell among us, to bring peace between God and man by saving our souls. Jesus came on earth to make that sacrifice by shedding His blood on the cross for the remission of our sins. He paid the penalty so that we can stand in His righteousness on the day that we die when we stand before the Holy God. By true repentance of our wrong doings and by putting our trust in Jesus and receiving Him as our Savior and Lord, we are redeemed and born of the Spirit. He is our Lord who reigns in our life. The missionaries greatly influenced the civilization and advancement of Hawaii. Rev. Bingham left Hawaii to go back home to New England in 1840.

The first Christian church built in Oahu was the Kawaiahao Church in downtown Honolulu across from the mission house. Construction took five years and more than a thousand men to build the church, made of coral reef rocks and an interior of wood from the Koolau Mountains. The church was dedicated in 1842 and is known as the Westminster Abbey of the Pacific. Many members of the Hawaiian royal family worshipped there. It is also where Rev. Dr. Judd, a medical missionary, read from the steps of the Church in 1843 the proclamation of the British Queen Victoria restoring Hawaii' sovereignty. The Hawaiian flag was raised again and King Kamehameha III proclaimed the motto *Ua mau ke ea o ka aina I ka pono*, which means "The life of the land is perpetuated in righteousness." Which is now the official motto. The mausoleum of King Lunalilo is on the church grounds, and a small cemetery is behind the church.

Weekly Sunday services are still performed at Kawaiahao Church.

Rev. Lorenzo Lyons, a protestant missionary, composed the hymn "I left It All With Jesus," the melody of which is now the popular Hawaiian song *"Hawaii Aloha"* that is performed as a stirring anthem after events.

Queen Kaahumanu who felt seriously ill was cared for and nursed by the wife of Rev. Bingham, Sybil. The queen got better and became attached to Christian teachings. The Queen had given her heart to Jesus and became a devout Christian and exercised her power for Protestant morality. She told the chiefs to instruct their people to observe the Sabbath day, attend school and church, as well as obey the Word of God. Prior to proclaiming the law against murder, theft and adultery by the Chiefs in 1827, Rev. Bingham was asked to review the law to make sure that it conformed with the Word of God. In 1829 she took a trip to Kona on the Big Island, to rebury the bones of the ancients chiefs. She also ordered couples in the islands to get married in a Christian ceremony. She traveled through Oahu to tell people the gospel of Jesus Christ and to worship the true God. In 1832, on her death bed she had sent for Rev. Bingham and before she peacefully died and went to be with the Lord, she whispered "Lo, here am I, O Jesus grant me thy gracious smile."

King Kauikeaouli was Kamehameha III. He ruled after the death of the Queen Kaahumanu. In 1843, he was challenged by Lord George Paulet, who anchored the Carysfort at Honolulu pressing the King to cede the kingdom to Britain. The troubled King had no way out and signed the papers. The Hawaiian flag was replaced for the British flag. Rev. Dr. Judd wrote an appeal on behalf of the King to the British Government, which prompted Admiral Sir Richard Thomas to sail to Honolulu to restore the sovereignty of Hawaii, five months later. In 1846, the King established the distribution of lands of Hawaii. Known as the Great Mahele. The King and his wife adopted a nephew Prince Alexander Liholiho who became the next king in 1854.

---

Moana took a break, chitchatted with the tourists, then continued with her stories.

---

Prince Alexander Liholiho was proclaimed King Kamehameha IV. He married Emma, a granddaughter of John Young. His close friend and minister of foreign affairs was a Scot, Robert Wyllie. Wyllie invested thousand of dollars in a coffee plantation in Hanalei on Kauai. After several years he changed the name to Princeville and started growing sugar.

King Lot Kamehameha V, the last Kamehameha, was proclaimed King in 1863. He died on his fortieth birthday in 1872. He was a bachelor and had not chosen a successor. King Lunalilo, half brother of Kamehameha the Great, was voted in by the members of the assembly and confirmed.

King William Lunalilo ruled briefly. Three of Lunalilo's four cabinet ministers were Americans. Lunalilo died in 1874 at the age of thirty-nine, without naming a successor to the throne. On his request he was put to rest at Kawaiahao Church instead of the royal mausoleum.

Both Kalakaua and Queen Emma began campaigning quietly for the throne. Emma was sure that she would win because she found Kalalaua to be an arrogant man inexperienced for the position and a big pretender. Kalakaua won the election by aggressive campaigning.

King Kalakaua made a trip to the United States in 1874. He was introduced to President Grant and was received by the houses of Congress in joint session in Washington. A state ball was given in his honor. Kalakaua signed a tax-free treaty with the United States, the so-called Reciprocity Treaty, in 1875.

He had the Iolani Palace built in downtown Honolulu, which was completed in 1882. Kalakaua formed a secret society, Hale Naua. The membership was limited to men with Hawaiian blood. A most devoted supporter of him was Walter Gibson, a political figure. He became his premier in 1882. Gibson supported a business man, Spreckels, who leased land from the government. Spreckels made the government an offer to get a fee, simple title for his twenty-four thousand acres of leased land on Maui. The bill was drawn up by Gibson and passed. Spreckelsville Sugar Plantation was founded in 1878. Spreckels partnered with Irwin and Company and controlled almost the entire Hawaiian sugar industry. The King was in debt to Spreckels. The King had to get a loan from a London Lender to pay off his debt to Spreckels. King Kalakaua and Gibson governed and made a mash-pash of the economy. When he died in 1891, his sister, Lydia, believed that her brother's early death was caused by his grief-stricken deeds. Lydia inherited the kingdom and was crowned Queen Liliuokalani. The last queen of Hawaii.

An American, Lorrin Thurston, a Protestant missionary grandson had formed with twelve men an Annexation Club, because they believed that good government would not be possible without an annexation with a powerful country.

The Queen was faced with a complex political situation. When the sugar industry was in trouble, the whole kingdom was in trouble. The Queen had her own ideas and ways to rule and wanted to proclaim her new constitution from the throne room and balcony; however, the ministers convinced her to postpone the proclamation. Her opponents felt that the time had come to take possession and proclaim a new regime. The Queen surrendered and was imprisoned in the Iolani Palace. She was released in 1895 and went back home to her house "Washington Palace" were she used to live with her husband, who was Governor of Oahu under King Lunalilo reign. Her beloved John Dominis, an American, had already passed away. Queen Liliuokalani had a talent for music and wrote beautiful Hawaiian songs, including the popular, beautiful farewell song *Aloha Oe*, which means *Farewell to thee*. She died at the age of seventy-nine. Liliuokalani Gardens, a thirty-acre park with beautiful flowers in Hilo, is dedicated to her.

The last princess was Hawaiians' favorite and beloved Victoria Kaiulani Cleghorn. She was born on October 16, 1875. Bells rang from church towers and the Hawaiians rejoiced. Her mother was Princess Likelike, the sister of King Kalakaua and Queen Liliuokalani, and her father was a wealthy Scot, Archibald Cleghorn who was the Oahu governor under Kalakaua's reign. He was also an expert in growing plants and flowers. On the grounds of the ten acres of land in Waikiki was their beautiful house with luscious gardens, palm trees, colorful tropical flowers and fruit trees. It was called Ainahau. Victoria enjoyed playing with and feeding her pets. She had peacocks and a turtle. She was a sweet, unspoiled, merry child who loved to ride her pony. Victoria was sadden by her mother's death. She was only twelve years old. Her dad sent her to England to school to prepare for her future royal duties since her aunt, Queen Liliuokalani had named her as successor. She lived in England for eight years. Before she returned home to Hawaii she visited the American President Grover Cleveland. She wanted to speak with him about Hawaii's annexation to America. In

Washington, she pleaded with him to save her kingdom from the annexation.

The princess became ill shortly after she returned to Hawaii and died on March 6, 1899, at the age of twenty-three. The Hawaiians were grief stricken; weeping they followed the hearse in the torch-lit procession that took her body from her home to the Kawaiahao Church where it laid for three days in state. Women were wailing songs. After three days laying in repose, a huge funeral took place. Cannons were fired and the honor guard carried the casket to the royal mausoleum in Nuuanu Valley, her final resting place. The royal kingdom of Hawaii ended with the death of the beautiful sweet princess.

---

Hawaii was made an United States territory in 1900 under President William McKinley. Military bases were established on the Hawaii Islands, including Pearl Harbor, a strategic important port, on Oahu. Congress allowed Hawaii's government to be replaced by a temporary government headed by Judge Sanford Dole.

"I hope that you enjoyed listening to my stories," said Moana with an emotion-filled voice She reached for the flower leis that she had next to her, and she gave her aloha and a lei to each tourist.

## The Land of Hawaii

The state of Hawaii, the Aloha state, is an archipelago consisting of eight islands in the Pacific Ocean. The islands, created by volcanic eruptions, are named and nicknamed: Ni'ihau (*The Forbidden Island*), Kaua'i (*The Garden Island*), O'ahu (*The Gathering Place*), Moloka'i (*The Friendly Island*), Lana'i (*The Pineapple Island*), Kaho'olawe (*The Forgotten Island*), Maui (*The Valley Island*), and Hawaii (*The Big Island*).

Hawaii has delicious fruits, awesome beaches, spectacular mountains, magnificent waterfalls, beautiful one of a kind flowers, plants, whales, dolphins and tropical colorful fish. It has a mild tropical climate; however, on the Big Island, snow covers the mountain of Mauna Kea and Mauna Loa. Experienced skiers can enjoy the ski slope in the morning and enjoy surfing in the afternoon. A native Hawaiian is a descendant of Polynesians (the aborigines). Hawaiians born on the islands could be Chinese (arrived in 1852), Japanese (arrived in 1885), Europeans, Filipinos, Americans, or Koreans descent Quite a rich blend of ethnicity. Hawaiian music, composed and arranged by many talented musicians, permeates throughout the islands. Luaus and hula dancing are still the favorite of the locals and tourists.

Now back to the diet!

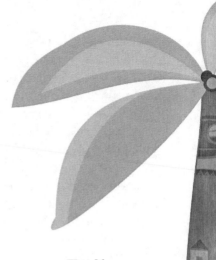

# Epilogue

My story was that I finally realized that food is to nourish the body so that the organs, cells, tissue, bones, muscle, and arteries can function properly. Food does taste good and should be enjoyed, not indulged.

I know how hard it can be to break the habit of overeating. One of the main reasons the eating cycle is not broken is that the mind tells us that being overweight is an acceptable way of life. Weight loss should be done by eating a well-balanced, healthy diet. We should become familiar with how the body functions and with the important role of fiber, vitamins, and minerals. Furthermore, we should become aware of the health effects of manmade toxins.

The key to permanent weight loss is eating in moderation; ingesting smaller portions; cutting fat, sugar, and carbohydrates; and making good nutritional choices. Exercise or brisk walking should be part of anybody's daily routine. Proper diet and exercise go hand in hand.

It was a pleasure taking you with me to Waikiki, Hawaii. If you need a weight loss goal, I suggest a trip to Hawaii. Remember, you are never alone on your journey. You have God Almighty whom you can call upon at any time.

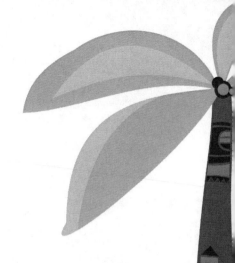

# Contact the Author

Marianne can be reached at waikikidiet@yahoo.com
Check out the Waikiki Diet on the web!
www.Waikikidiet.com

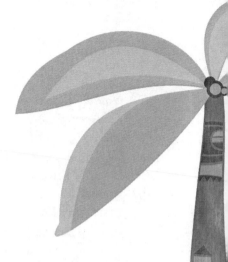

# Notes

## Waikiki

[1] Dukes' Canoe Club–a restaurant at the Outrigger Hotel, Waikiki

[2] Hula Girl–a restaurant at the Outrigger Hotel, Waikiki

## First Things First

[1] Exercise–Dr. Colbert, MD, *Seven Pillars of Health*, Siloam, Lake Mary, FL., Chapter: The Benefits of Exercise, page 119, 123

## Six Day Diet

[1] Decaf coffee–William Manahan, MD, *Eat for Health*, HJ Kramer Inc., Tiburon, CA Chapter: A simple Test, page 34

[2] Caffeine–William Manahan, MD, *Eat for Health*, HJ Kramer, Inc., Tiburon, CA, Chapter: The Harmful Effects of Caffeine, page 8

[3] Mrs. Mango's Hibiscus Flower Herb Tea, Mrs. Mango's Herbs Etc., Rockledge, FL, 321-631-1194, The tea is made of Wild Hibiscus flowers, Rosehips, Lemon balm, Orange peel and Mint.

[4] Vitamin C–Don Colbert, MD, *Toxic Relief*, Siloam, Lake Mary, FL, Chapter: The Joy of Juice, pages 73, 67 and Don Colbert, MD, *Living in Divine Health* page 21, 22

[5] Enzymes–Don Colbert MD, *Living in Divine Health*, Siloam, Lake Mary, FL, topic: Enzymes, page 39, 40

## Protein, Fiber, Fat, Salt, Sugar and the Glycemic Index

[1] Protein-Linda Clark, MA., *Know Your Nutrition*, Keats Publishing, Inc., New Canaan, CT, chapter: Protein, the Real Staff of Life, page 236, 237

3 Excess protein–Don Colbert MD, *The Seven Pillars of Health*, Siloam, Lake Mary, FL, Chapter: What to eat With Caution-Meat and Dairy, page 102

4 Fiber –Don Colbert MD, *Toxic Relief*, Siloam, Lake Mary, FL, Chapter: Eliminate the Negative, pages 152,153

5 Fiber–Don Colbert MD, *The Seven Pillars of Health*, Siloam, Lake Mary, FL, Chapter: What to Avoid the Dark Side of the Food World, page 93

6 Gallbladder–Linda Clark, MA, *Know Your Nutrition*, Keats Publishing, Inc., New Canaan, CT, Chapter: Cholesterol, Fats and Oils, page 205

7 Fat–Don Colbert MD, The Seven Pillars of Health, Siloam, Lake Mary, FL., Chapter: What to Avoid-the Dark Side of the Food World, pages 87, 88,89

8 Extracting oil–Linda Clark, MA, *Know Your Nutrition*, Keats Publishing, Inc., New Canaan, CT, chapter: Cholesterol, Fats and Oils, page 209

9 Salt–William Manahan, MD, *Eat for Health*, HJ Kramer, Inc., Tiburon, CA, Chapter: The Effectsof Too Much Salt, page 38

10 Heart–William Manahan, MD, *Eat for Health*, HJ Kramer, Inc., Tiburon, CA, Chapter: The Effects of Too Much Salt, page 39

11 Sugar–Don Colbert, MD, *The Seven Pillars of*

*Health*, Siloam, Lake Mary, FL., Chapter: What to Avoid-the Dark Side of the Food World, page 80

[12] Dopamine–Don Colbert, MD, *The Seven Pillars of Health*, Siloam, Lake Mary, FL, Chapter: Your Body is a Temple, page 69

## Toxins & Nutrients

[13] Pesticide residues–Don Colbert, MD, *The Seven Pillars of Health*, Siloam, Lake Mary, FL, Chapter: What to eat With Caution-Meat and Dairy, page 107

[14] MSG–Don Colbert, MD, *The Seven Pillars of Health*, Siloam, Lake Mary, FL, Chapter: What to Avoid-the Dark Side of the Food World, page 77

[15] Processed food–Don Colbert MD, *The Seven Pillars of Health*, Siloam, Lake Mary, FL, Chapter: What to Avoid-the Dark Side of the Food World, page 77

[16] Toxins in fat–Don Colbert, MD, *The Seven Pillars of Health*, Siloam, Lake Mary, FL, Chapter: What to eat With Caution-Meat and Dairy, page 101

[17] Second hand smoke–Don Colbert MD, *Living in Divine Health*, Lake Mary, FL., Topic: Lung Cancer, page 10

[18] Cigarettes–Don Colbert, MD, *Toxic Relief*, Siloam, Lake Mary, FL., chapter: Our Toxin Earth, pages 12, 67

[19] Free radicals–Don Colbert, MD, *The Seven Pillars of Health*, Siloam, Lake Mary, FL, Chapter: Your Need for Antioxidants, pages 198,199

[20] The liver–Don Colbert, MD, *Toxic Relief*, Siloam, Lake Mary, FL, Chapter: Your Champion Prize Fighter, pages 105, 106

[21] Antioxidants–Don Colbert MD, *The Seven Pillars of Health*, Siloam, Lake Mary, FL ,Chapter: Your need for Antioxidants, page 202

[22] Phytonutrients–Don Colbert MD, *The Seven Pillars of Health*, Siloam, Lake Mary, FL, Chapter: The Power of Phytonutrients, page 205

## Supplements & Maintenance

[1] Supplements–Don Colbert MD, *The Seven Pillars of Health*, Siloam, Lake Mary, FL, Chapter: How to pick the Right Supplements, page 222 to 227

[2] Lecithin–Linda Clark, MA., *Know Your Nutrition*, Keats Publishing, Inc., New Canaan, CT, Chapter: High Power Foods, page 216

## Waikiki, Captain Cook and Hawaiian Royalty

[1] Moana story–bibliography Captain Cook and Hawaiian Royalty

[2] Shoal of Time, A history of the Hawaiian Islands by Gaven Daws, The MacMillan Company, New York

[3] The Last Princess, The story of Princess Kaiulani of Hawaii by Fay Stanley, Four Winds Press, Macmillan International Publishing Group, New York

[4] The last Hawaiian Queen Liliuokalani by Paula Guzzetti, Benchmark Books, Marshall Cavendish, New York

# Shopping List

| # | Shopping List | Store | Notes |
|---|---|---|---|
| | | | |
| | **Grains:** | | |
| | Whole grain bread | | |
| | Kavli crisp bread | | |
| | Nature's Path, flax plus multibran cereal | | |
| | Whole grain pasta | | |
| | | | |
| | **Diary :** | | |
| | Egg Whites | | |
| | Egg beater | | |
| | Organic brown eggs | | |
| | Yogurt, organic, fat free | | |
| | Cheese slices, fat free | | |
| | Laughing Cow light cheese | | |
| | White Cheese sticks, low or fat free | | |
| | Half-and-half, fat free | | |
| | Half-and-half, organic | | |
| | Milk, fat free (skim) | | |
| | Milk, organic, fat free | | |
| | | | |
| | **Oils :** | | |
| | Virgin Olive Oil, organic | | |
| | Sesame Oil | | |
| | Flax Seed oil | | |
| | | | |

| | | | |
|---|---|---|---|
| | **Herbs/spices :** | | |
| | Montreal steak spices | | |
| | Garlic Powder | | |
| | Onion Powder | | |
| | Rosemary | | |
| | | | |
| | **Vegetables :** | | |
| | Romaine lettuce | | |
| | asparagus | | |
| | beans | | |
| | bean sprouts – organic | | |
| | bell peppers | | |
| | brocolli | | |
| | cabbage | | |
| | carrots | | |
| | cucumber | | |
| | onions | | |
| | spinach | | |
| | squash | | |
| | sweet potato | | |
| | tomatoes | | |
| | zuchinni | | |
| | | | |
| | **Fruits :** | | |
| | apples | | |
| | avocado | | |
| | bananas | | |
| | berries | | |

| | | |
|---|---|---|
| mandarin | | |
| orange | | |
| papaya | | |
| pineapple | | |
| water melon | | |
| | | |
| Dried organic fruits | | |
| Frozen organic berries | | |
| | | |
| **Legumes :** | | |
| Red Kidney beans | | |
| Navy beans | | |
| Pinto beans | | |
| Black beans | | |
| | | |
| **Meat :** | | |
| Natural Chicken Breast fillets | | |
| Turkey Breast | | |
| Steak | | |
| Pork | | |
| | | |
| **Fish & Seafood :** | | |
| orange roughy | | |
| salmon | | |
| shrimps | | |
| snapper | | |
| tilapia | | |
| | | |

| | | | |
|---|---|---|---|
| | **Other :** | | |
| | Almonds, sliced | | |
| | Coffee, decaf | | |
| | Dark Chocolate | | |
| | Flax seed, ground | | |
| | Fruit popsicle | | |
| | Green tea | | |
| | Herbal tea | | |
| | Roasted soy bean nuts | | |
| | Salad Dressing, Newman's Own | | |
| | V8 | | |
| | Walnuts | | |
| | Water | | |
| | | | |